CONTRIBUTORS

Scope and Standards Workgroup

Karen E. Greco, PhD, RN, ANP
Cynthia A. Prows, MSN, RN
Heather Skirton, PhD, RN, Certified Midwife, Registered Genetic
  Counsellor (UK)
Janet Williams, PhD, RN, CPNP, Certified Genetic Counselor
Shirley Jones, PhD, RNC, Certified Genetic Counselor
Lindsay Middelton, RN, Certified Genetic Counselor
Judith Lewis, PhD, RNC, FAAN

ANA Staff

Carol J. Bickford, PhD, RN, BC
Yvonne Daley Humes, MSA
Matthew Seiler, RN, Esq.

Winifred Carson-Smith, JD—Consultant

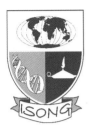

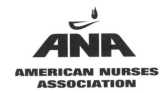

AMERICAN NURSES
ASSOCIATION

GENETICS/GENOMICS NURSING:

SCOPE AND STANDARDS

OF PRACTICE

nurses
books
.org

The Publishing Program of ANA

AMERICAN NURSES ASSOCIATION
SILVER SPRING, MARYLAND
2007

Library of Congress Cataloging-in-Publication data

International Society of Nurses in Genetics.
   Genetics/genomics nursing : scope and standards of practice / International Society of Nurses in Genetics and American Nurses Association.
      p. ; cm.
   Includes bibliographical references and index.
   ISBN-13: 978-1-55810-234-7 (pbk.)
   ISBN-10: 1-55810-234-5 (pbk.)
      1. Genetic disorders—Nursing—Standards.   2. Medical genetics.   3. Genetic counseling.   4. Nursing—Standards.   I. American Nurses Association.   II. Title.
      [DNLM: 1. Specialties, Nursing—standards.   2. Nurse's Role.   3. Nursing Care—standards. WY 16 I618g 2006]

RB155.5.I555 2006
   616'.042—dc22   2006028823

The American Nurses Association (ANA) is a national professional association. This ANA publication—*Genetics/Genomics Nursing: Scope and Standards of Practice*—reflects the thinking of the nursing profession on various issues and should be reviewed in conjunction with state board of nursing policies and practices. State law, rules, and regulations govern the practice of nursing, while *Genetics/Genomics Nursing: Scope and Standards of Practice* guides nurses in the application of their professional skills and responsibilities.

Published by Nursesbooks.org
The Publishing Program of ANA

American Nurses Association
8515 Georgia Avenue, Suite 400
Silver Spring, MD 20910-3492
1-800-274-4ANA
http://www.nursesbooks.org/

ANA is the only full-service professional organization representing the nation's 2.7 million Registered Nurses through its 54 constituent member associations. ANA advances the nursing profession by fostering high standards of nursing practice, promoting the economic and general welfare of nurses in the workplace, projecting a positive and realistic view of nursing, and lobbying the Congress and regulatory agencies on healthcare issues affecting nurses and the public.

The International Society of Nurses in Genetics (ISONG) is a global nursing specialty organization dedicated to fostering the scientific and professional growth of nurses in human genetics and genomics worldwide. The ISONG vision is: Caring for people's genetic and genomic health.

Design: Scott Bell & Stacy Maguire ~ *Composition*: House of Equations, Inc. ~ *Copyediting*: Steven Jent & Lisa Anthony ~ *Indexing*: Steven Jent ~ *Printing*: McArdle Printing

First printing October 2006.

ISBN-13: 978-1-55810-234-7   ISBN-10: 1-55810-234-5   SAN: 851-3481
06SSGG   2M   10/06

CONTENTS

Scope of Genetics/Genomics Nursing Practice

The International Society of Nurses in Genetics (ISONG) has a diverse membership befitting its name. ISONG is the official professional organization of nurses in genetics in the United States, and also represents genetics nurses worldwide. This document therefore applies to genetics nursing in many different national contexts.

ISONG is responsible for defining and establishing the scope of professional nursing practice in genetics for nurses globally. ISONG acknowledges the role of the American Nurses Association (ANA) in defining the scope of practice for the nursing profession as a whole in the United States and supports the ANA *Social Policy Statement* (2003), which charges specialty nursing organizations with defining their individual scopes of practice and identifying the unique characteristics of their specialties. In keeping with ISONG's responsibility, this document broadly describes genetics and genomics nursing practice, then delineates the scope of genetics clinical nursing practice in the United States. ISONG and ANA recognize that this document may be adopted globally.

Interaction of Genetics and Genomics

The Human Genome Project has laid the foundation for enormous advances in the fields of genetics and genomics. In response, genetics nursing practice has evolved significantly since the publication of ISONG's scope and standards of genetics clinical nursing practice in 1998. Research efforts are improving our understanding of the functions and interactions of all genes in the human genome as well as interactions with environmental factors. This genetic revolution has resulted in a paradigm shift from genetics to genomics, which is much broader and affects all areas of nursing practice. *Genomics* refers to the study of all the genes in the human genome together, including their interactions with each other and the environment. *Genetics* refers to the examination and understanding of genes and their effects. The ability to understand the role of genetics in human health and disease is a tremendous step toward better prevention, treatment, and potentially cures for common diseases and health problems (Guttmacher, Collins, & Drazen, 2004).

Scientific discoveries are enhancing clinical capabilities in diagnosing and treating rare single-gene disorders. Likewise, advancements further the ability to predict susceptibility to and promote preventive therapies for genetically influenced chronic conditions such as cardiovascular and autoimmune diseases, cancer, and diabetes. Genetic and genomic investigation of infectious diseases, once thought impracticable, has increased the speed of diagnosis, the effectiveness of existing therapies, and the development of new therapies. This expanding knowledge will continue to affect how genetics and genomics services are defined and delivered. These services extend into an increasing variety of settings. Clinical genetics services include:

- providing genetics and genomics services to individuals, families, groups, communities, and populations,

- providing and managing comprehensive care, which includes state-of-the-art genetics screening, diagnosis, counseling, and therapeutic modalities,

- evaluating and improving genetics and genomics services,

- educating individuals, families, and public and professional populations about genetics and genomics, and

- assessing, deliberating, and developing recommendations for ethical, legal, and social consequences of new and existing genetics and genomics services and technology.

Definition of Genetics/Genomics Nursing

Genetics/genomics nursing is the protection, promotion, and optimization of health and abilities, prevention of illness and injury, alleviation of suffering through the diagnosis of human response, and advocacy in the care of the genetic and genomic health of individuals, families, communities, and populations. This includes health issues, genetic conditions, and diseases or susceptibilities to diseases caused or influenced by genes in interaction with other risk factors that may require nursing care.

Genetics nursing has traditionally involved the care of people with single-gene and chromosome disorders such as cystic fibrosis, Huntington disease, and Down syndrome. However, even single-gene disorders are modified by other genes and the environment, thus broadening the nursing specialty to include genomics nursing, which involves health issues related to multiple genes in the human genome, including their interactions with each other and the environment, and the influence of other psychosocial and cultural factors.

The term *genetics nursing* is still primarily used throughout this document because:

- nurses, physicians, and counselors in this specialty use "genetic" or "genetics" in their professional titles;

- certifying boards in this field award "genetic(s)" credentials; and

- national and international organizations representing the majority of professionals in this field still use "genetic" or "genetics" in their names.

The International Evolution of Genetics/Genomics Nursing Practice

Contemporary genetics and genomics nursing practice builds on decades of work by nurses and others in the United States, Canada, Japan, the United Kingdom, and several other countries. While such work is by its nature interdependent, it is more conveniently described nation by nation.

United States

Genetics nursing practice in the United States has its historical roots in public health nursing, prenatal and neonatal screening, and pediatrics. Nurses in these specialties were among the first healthcare professionals to provide care for and address the needs of individuals and families diagnosed with or at risk for transmission of a genetic condition. Historically, genetics services were often provided by public health nurses through maternal and child health programs. In the 1960s, nurses in North America and Europe began to describe the implications of genetics for professional practice and the care of individuals, families, and communities.

In the United States, the passage of the Genetic Diseases Act in 1976 and the subsequent funding of state and federal programs to provide prenatal and pediatric genetics services (under the aegis of the Public Health Service) brought the importance of integrating genetics into clinical nursing practice to the attention of nurse clinicians, administrators, researchers, and academicians. A landmark consensus conference was held in 1980 to identify the current level of genetics education received by undergraduate and graduate nurses, to describe the genetics knowledge needed by all nurses, and to make recommendations for programs to address the gaps between knowledge and practice (Forsman, 1994). Between 1980 and 1984, a growing number of nurses participated in local, state, and federal genetics services programs. Activities included the development of collegiate and continuing education genetics programs for nurses, facilitation of community support groups for individuals or families confronted with or at risk for a genetic disorder, and support of public policy on behalf of those individuals and families. In 1982 the first genetic nurses were certified as genetic counselors by the American Board of Medical Genetics. Eligibility requirements for certification as a genetic counselor were later changed; currently only nurses who have a master's degree in genetic counseling are eligible to sit for the required examination for certification as a genetic counselor.

The Genetic Nurses Network, formed in 1984, brought together for the first time nurses who identified their practice as genetics nursing. Educational programs that highlighted the unique aspects of genetics nursing practice within the broader scope of professional nursing advanced the professional development of these nurses. Originally, nurses came to this specialty with undergraduate and graduate degrees in nursing and clinical expertise in maternal–child, pediatric, and women's health nursing. As knowledge of human genetics advanced, so did the breadth and diversity of nurses who identified their primary practice as genetics nursing. Nurses with clinical expertise in the neurosciences, oncology, adult complex disorders, and behavioral sciences increasingly integrated the scientific and technologic advances into their practice with brought about by the Human Genome Research Initiative.

The International Society of Nurses in Genetics (ISONG) was established in 1988 to foster the scientific, professional and personal development of genetics nurses worldwide in the management of genetic information. ISONG's original vision, "Caring for people's genetic health," has changed little in their current vison, "Caring for people's genetic and genomic health." Throughout the 1990s, nurse clinicians and researchers

continued to define the requisite knowledge and the scope of genetics nursing practice. In 1997 ANA conferred specialty practice status on
genetics nursing in the United States. This was followed by the initial
publication of the scope and standards of clinical genetics nursing
practice (ISONG & ANA, 1998). ISONG recognized that genetics nurses
needed credentialing in order to establish genetics competency and
created a formal credentialing committee in 1999. Working from
the ISONG scope and standards of genetics nursing practice, the
credentialing committee compiled a list of core competencies and assessment measures for credentialing genetics nurses at the baccalaureate and master's level (Cook, Kase, Middelton, & Monsen, 2003). In 2002,
the Genetic Nursing Credentialing Commission (GNCC) was created
separate from ISONG to oversee the credentialing of nurses in genetics
(Monsen, 2005).

Canada

Genetics nursing practice in Canada evolved as in the United States, with
roots in obstetrics, neonatology and pediatrics. Medical genetics centers
provided genetics counseling as early as the 1970s. As these early genetics centers were established, the great majority of non-physician
counseling staff consisted of nurses from those specialties and a few
other healthcare workers such as social workers and people with a science degree in genetics. These became the first "genetics counselors,"
providing information and support for families with genetics concerns.
All genetics centers at this time were associated with hospital-based
university departments.

Although the Canadian College of Medical Geneticists defined strict
standards of practice, credentialing, and formalized training, there was
no training or credentialing for nurses and the other counselors other
than learning on the job and attending courses and in-services when
possible. The obvious need for standardized training led to the formation of three Master of Genetic Counseling programs across the coun-
try. The next step was the organization of the Canadian Association of
Genetic Counselors (CAGC) in 1990. CAGC became the credentialing
body for genetic counselors. Concerns about specific training for each
group of professionals (nurses, genetic counselors from the master's
programs, social workers, and those with a science degree in genetics)
have made it difficult to agree on common certification, thus impeding
the unique collaboration between these groups.

There is still no genetics training specifically for nurses in Canada, other than a variety of undergraduate and graduate university science courses available as electives, or through the U.S. or Canadian Master in Genetic Counseling programs. The three Canadian programs are unable to accept the numbers of applicants requesting admission, and funding for the counseling positions needed in the community continues to fluctuate. As more genetics counselors graduate from the Canadian and U.S. programs, fewer nurses are offered positions in genetics departments unless they have certification from CAGC. In addition, stringent CAGC requirements discourage many practicing nurses from becoming certified in genetics.

The need for genetics services in the different medical specialties is increasingly recognized. There is a movement to collaborate with departments of genetics, faculties of nursing, and the different medical specialties to offer nurses genetics training. Many provinces have Public Health Nurses associated with the genetics departments in the major centers, who are dedicated to providing genetics information, support, and services to rural areas. Genetics services in Canada are provided under the Health Care budget, and therefore individuals are not billed for services.

Increased awareness of the contribution of nurses to genetics health care in training institutions, and now the credentialing of nurses through the Genetic Nursing Credentialing Commission (GNCC), may prompt the Canadian Nurses Association to recognize genetics nursing as a specialty and bring more recognition to the field of genetics nursing in Canada.

Japan

Genetics nursing practice in Japan has its historical roots in public health nursing. Community nurses were among the first healthcare professionals to provide care for and address the needs of those found to have or be at risk for conditions or diseases with a genetic component. After World War II, new nursing legislation gave nurses three possible professional titles: Nurse, Nurse-Midwife, and Public Health Nurse. Genetic counseling was provided primarily in health centers in the community. Public Health Nurses identified and followed clients affected by genetic anomalies, conditions, or diseases through home visiting.

The Genetic Nursing Committee of Japan was established in 1999, bringing together for the first time nurses whose practice centered on genetics nursing. A study of the current level of genetics education received by undergraduate and graduate nurses described the genetics knowledge needed by all nurses and recommended the creation of programs to close the gaps between knowledge and practice (Arimori et al., 2000). Core competencies in genetics were then identified, developed, and implemented into nursing education programs (Ando, 2001; Mizoguchi et al., 2002). A landmark conference in 2001 formulated the ethics of nursing practice in genetics at the Japan Academy of Nursing Science (Ando, Takeda, & Williams, 2001). The Genetic Nursing Committee of Japan planned educational programs for the unique aspects of genetics nursing practice and the professional development of Japanese genetics nurses starting in 2001. Participants in this program had undergraduate and graduate degrees in nursing and clinical expertise in maternal–child, pediatric, and women's health nursing, oncology, and adult complex disorders (Mizoguchi et al., 2002; Morita et al., 2003). Additionally, continuing education programs for basic genetics nursing in the Japan Nurses Association will be operational from 2005. The first graduate program for genetics nursing in Japan was launched in 2005 at Tokai University (Mizoguchi, 2004).

In 2001 the Genetic Nursing Committee of Japan organized the first annual conference for genetics nursing to foster the scientific, professional, and personal development of members in the management of genetic information and support of genetics nursing practice.

United Kingdom

Genetics nurses from the United Kingdom have been at the forefront of developments in the care of clients affected by genetic disease. Clinical genetics developed as a specialty in health care in the United Kingdom alongside that in the United States, and was established as a clinical service in the years following the Second World War. Genetics nurses play a significant role in the provision of these services, usually working in teams with medical colleagues.

All genetics services in the UK are provided by the National Health Service, and clients are therefore not billed for their care. Genetics nurses have traditionally provided psychological support for clients and supported the work of medical colleagues before, during, and after clinic appointments. Increasingly they are accountable for their own caseload and work autonomously within the team (Skirton, Barnes, Curtis, &

Walford-Moore, 1997; Skirton et al., 1998). The professional organization, the Association of Genetic Nurses and Counsellors (AGNC) (www.agnc.org.uk), has been active for over 20 years; through the work of an Education Working Group, it introduced a registration system in 2001, although nursing practice is also governed by statutory regulation (Education Working Group of the AGNC, 2001; Skirton et al., 2003). Assessment of fitness to practice as a genetics nurse is based on a portfolio of evidence (including case log book, case studies, and supervisor's reports) submitted to the AGNC Registration Board. A recent white paper (Department of Health, 2003) emphasized that specialists in genetics health care must be appropriately educated, and endorsed the registration system introduced by the AGNC.

Other Countries

In Belgium, Australia, New Zealand, and the Netherlands, the contribution of nurses to specialist genetics health care is well established, while in Brazil, Israel, and Italy the role of genetics nurses is emerging through the efforts of nursing leadership. A formal registration procedure for genetics nurses in the Netherlands is managed by the Vereniging Klinische Geneticia Nederland (http://www.nav-vkgn.nl/).

A global professional framework is needed to ensure the safe and competent practice of genetics nurses. In the United States, Canada, the United Kingdom, and the Netherlands this has been addressed, but general standards of practice are needed to provide a foundation for safe nursing care. Different legal systems and educational structures in different countries make standardization of practice through academic assessment difficult. Setting standards of genetics clinical nursing practice would enable nurses from many nations to establish requisite levels of competence and relevant means of assessment for professional practice in their own setting.

Description of Genetics/Genomics Nursing

The genetics nursing specialty focuses on providing client-centered nursing care, education, or research based on understanding the underlying genetics and genomics of the individuals, families, communities, or populations affected by, or at risk for, diseases or conditions with a genetic component. Genetics nursing practice strives to be evidence-based. Genetic conditions are anomalies, behaviors, diseases, issues, or predispositions caused or influenced by genes which may affect one's health or abilities and may or may not be inherited. Genetics nursing practice includes genomics, which encompasses all the genes in the human genome together, including their interactions with each other and the environment, and the implications for health and nursing care. For the purpose of this document, the term *genetic conditions* will also include congenital anomalies, which may be the result of a genetic alteration or abnormal embryonic development and can range from minor to severe, resulting in anomalies, debilitating disease, a physical or mental disability, or premature death.

Genetics nursing practice may occur in any setting. Genetics nursing involves a personal relationship between client and nurse. Recipients of genetics nursing practice may be individuals, families, communities, or populations including but not limited to:

- people in any stage of life (from birth to death) who have a genetic condition,
- presymptomatic persons and families at risk for an inherited genetic condition,
- people susceptible to diseases which have a genetic component,
- couples at risk for having a child with a genetic condition, and
- people who need or request genetic information.

Comprehensive genetics nursing practice is a dynamic process. It involves interdisciplinary collegiality and collaboration with genetics professionals and other healthcare professionals to serve a shared mission of helping individuals, families, communities, or populations reach their desired health outcomes.

In this document the term *client* will be used instead of *patient* to refer to the recipient(s) of nursing services. *Patient* may have a connotation of illness, and in genetics nursing practice the recipients of nursing services include individuals, families, communities, and populations with, or at risk for, a genetic condition. In addition, in the education setting *client* includes the students being taught, while in research *client* includes participants in the research setting.

Essential Attributes of Genetics/Genomics Nursing

The four essential features of genetics nursing practice are:

1. Attention to the full range of human experiences and responses to the health and illness of clients related to discovery of and experiences with health issues related to genetics and genomics.

2. Application of genetics knowledge to the processes of nursing care, education, and research related to:

   - health education, promotion, maintenance, and restoration, optimization of health and abilities, prevention of illness and injury, alleviation of suffering, or a peaceful death;

   - making informed decisions related to genetic conditions or diseases and the use of available genetic technology and services; and

   - participation in a complex healthcare system.

3. Integration of objective data with knowledge gained from an understanding of the client's subjective experience with or risk of a genetic condition or a chronic disease that has a genetic component and associated disability or morbidity.

4. A caring relationship that facilitates health and healing and considers the ethical, legal, and social issues associated with a genetic condition, genetic susceptibility to a disease, or malformation.

Genetics nursing is built on a body of knowledge that comprises the dual components of science and art. It is a scientific discipline as well as a profession. Genetics nursing uses a number of theories for assessing, diagnosing, planning, implementing, and evaluating care that is responsive to the essential attributes of genetics nursing practice. Such theories are derived from nursing, genetic, biological, behavioral, social, and medical sciences as well as other related fields. These theories provide a framework for understanding, implementing, and evaluating the practice of genetics nurses.

The International Council of Nurses' *Code of Ethics for Nurses* (2001) is the standard for ethical nursing practice worldwide. *Code of Ethics for Nurses with Interpretive Statements* (ANA, 2001) and similar ethical guidelines provide a framework to guide ethical nursing practice in the United

States and worldwide. Sensitivity to cultural, lifestyle, racial, and ethnic diversity is integral to planning and providing services for clients with genetic conditions. The central axiom of the profession is respect for individuals, and in this context the nurse supports the client's self-determination and autonomy.

Practice Settings

Genetics nurses practice in healthcare settings that include but are not limited to: hospitals and their affiliated clinics, academic medical centers and universities; regional genetic centers; ambulatory and primary healthcare facilities; industrial, community and school health settings; state and federal agencies; private industry (including clinical and biotechnology laboratories and pharmaceutical companies); managed healthcare organizations; and healthcare recipient and provider insurance organizations. As genetic services continue to expand into a variety of settings, especially primary care settings, so too will genetics nursing practice.

- A school nurse trained in genetics consoles a student who tearfully reveals her father died from sudden bleeding in his chest. The information causes the school nurse to reassess the adolescent's tall stature and long extremities—rather than volleyball assets, the features could be part of Marfan syndrome. The school nurse calls the adolescent's mother to obtain more information and discuss her concern and the possibility of a genetics referral.

- Genetics nurses practicing in specialty clinics that focus on single-gene disorders such as cystic fibrosis, sickle cell, and hemophilia may provide care to their specialty population that includes providing information about the relevant inheritance pattern, genetic testing, and implications of test results.

- Genetics nurses in advanced practice working at regional genetics centers in an academic affiliated medical center may evaluate, diagnose, counsel, and manage clients with or at risk for a genetic condition. Most genetics nurses in advanced practice focus on the genetics needs of specific patient populations rather than all patients who enter the genetics center. They are often part of an interdisciplinary team of genetics professionals, and their actual roles and responsibilities are often influenced by the expertise and practice of other team members.

- Genetics nurse entrepreneurs in advanced practice may market their expertise to managed care and insurance organizations to help their staff evaluate the clinical utility of various genetic tests and differentiate between dubious predisposition tests being marketed directly to consumers for unproven purposes—such as skin creams and nutritional supplements—and predisposition genetic tests backed by scientific evidence. Genetics APNs can also substantiate the types and levels of services that may be needed for specific genetic tests, such as genetics counseling needed before and after testing for Huntington disease but unnecessary for pharmacogenetic testing prior to prescribing a medication.

Levels of Genetics/Genomics Nursing Practice

The scope of genetics specialty nursing practice comprises two levels: basic and advanced. Both include application of genetics and genomics knowledge in risk assessment, outcome identification, intervention, and evaluation. What distinguishes them is the depth and breadth of knowledge and skills. For example, a forty-year-old adult female with a family history of breast cancer is being evaluated as a new client. The genetics nurse practicing at the basic level applies fundamental genetics knowledge in conducting a cancer risk assessment that encompasses environmental and genetics components. The genetics nurse collects and records a family pedigree, identifies components of the family history that may suggest the woman may be at risk for an inherited form of breast or ovarian cancer, explains this potential risk to the client, develops a referral plan with the client, facilitates a referral to a genetics nurse in advanced practice, provides psychosocial support, evaluates the interventions, and assesses the client's understanding and ability to implement a plan of surveillance or treatment following the referral.

The genetics nurse in advanced practice conducts a more thorough cancer risk assessment with interpretation of familial and other risk factors, provides comprehensive, balanced information about predisposition genetic testing for breast or ovarian cancer to enable the woman to make an informed decision about testing, discusses interpretation of genetic test results with the client, determines her need of assistance in communicating test results with the family, discusses surveillance and cancer risk-reduction options, develops a plan with the client, facilitates communication with the client, family, and other care providers, evaluates the client's plan of care, and monitors outcomes of the interventions.

These levels of practice are distinguished by educational preparation, professional experience, practice focus, specific roles and functions, and specialty certification or credentialing. Professional nursing colleagues and professional regulatory organizations ensure that nursing practice is within the legal framework and follows practice standards.

Basic Level

Basic level genetics nurses routinely provide genetics services to clients. They are expected to have either formal genetics clinical experiences from their basic nursing preparatory programs or on-the-job training from professionals trained in genetics such as graduate nursing or medical faculty with genetics expertise, advanced practice nurses in a genetics healthcare setting, appropriately credentialed genetics professionals, or other clinicians who provide genetics-based clinical services or conduct genetic research within their specialty.

The genetics nurse's knowledge and skill base is maintained through participation in genetics and nursing continuing education. Credentialing in genetics is strongly encouraged.

Advanced Level

The characteristics that distinguish advanced from basic level genetics nursing practice are expanded practice skills and knowledge in nursing and genetics, increased complexity of decision-making, leadership, and the ability to negotiate complex organizations. Throughout this document, a nurse with a graduate degree in nursing who practices in genetics at the advanced practice level will be referred to as a *genetics nurse in advanced practice*.

Genetics nurses in advanced practice are nurses who have successfully completed an accredited graduate (master's or doctoral) program in nursing and routinely provide genetics services to clients. They are expected to have completed a genetics curriculum that includes human, molecular, biochemical, and population genetics, technological applications, therapeutic modalities, and ethical, legal, and social implications of genetics information and technology. They are also expected to have either formal genetics clinical experiences or on-the-job training in their specified advanced practice role under the supervision of a professional trained in genetics.

The genetics nurse in advanced practice is expected to maintain their knowledge and skill base through ongoing participation in genetics and nursing continued education. This knowledge can be acquired through completion of didactic and clinical courses in a formal program of study leading to a master's or doctoral degree in nursing with a concentration in advanced practice in genetics nursing. Didactic or clinical courses may also be obtained through postgraduate degree certification programs.

Nurses may achieve a PhD in Nursing or a related discipline, or a practice doctorate that includes academic courses focused on specific clinical or research genetics content. Credentialing in genetics at the advanced practice level is strongly encouraged.

In the United States, *advanced practice registered nurse* or APRN refers to a registered nurse with a master's or doctoral degree practicing as a nurse practitioner (NP), clinical nurse specialist (CNS), certified nurse midwife (CNM), or certified registered nurse anesthetist (CRNA). In addition, U.S. nurses who prepare to be Advanced Practice Registered Nurses (APRNs) must also complete academic or continuing education courses as specified by state and national organizations that set standards for advanced practice licensure. Outside the United States, *advanced practice nurse* is the term most widely used when referring to advanced practice roles.

The original scope and standards of clinical genetics nursing practice focused on traditional advanced practice roles such as NP, CNS, CNM, and CRNA, consistent with the definition of advanced practice registered nursing for these four roles (ISONG & ANA, 1998). Although CRNAs do not typically practice in genetics settings, the standards offer guidance in those areas where genetics bears on CRNA practice. For example, pharmacogenetics and polymorphisms related to drug uptake, metabolism, and excretion are critical to CRNA practice.

These traditional roles for genetics nurses in advanced practice have evolved to include research, education, and administration in a wide variety of clinical arenas. At the same time genetics nurses with advanced nursing degrees are using their advanced practice skills in ways that affect the genomic health of individuals, families, communities, and populations through research, education, policy, administration, and other activities. Technological advances have also expanded clinical nursing practice to include health care provided through telemedicine, computerized patient education, and interactive technology. As a result, contemporary genetics/genomics nursing practice is broad and diverse. The scope and standards of genetics and genomics nursing practice uses the term *genetics nurses in advanced practice* which is intended to include the broad range of genetics nurse advanced practice roles.

Genetic conditions affect a significant portion of the general population, although any one condition is relatively rare. People with a genetic condition may require health and social services from a number of professionals, depending on the types of problems caused by the condition. While most of those providing care may focus on a system or type of problem, the genetics nurse is able to address the impact of the condition as a whole and the issues that arise from the potentially inherited nature of the condition. Furthermore, the genetics nurse offers holistic family care that addresses the needs of the affected individuals, family members at risk for the condition, carriers, and parents of affected children.

A Case Study in Genetics/Genomics Nursing Practice

Suppose Tom is 25 years old and has two young children. He is referred to a genetics nurse in advanced practice by his family doctor after he expresses concerns about his mother's recent diagnosis of colon cancer. The genetics nurse in advanced practice collects a family history and learns that Tom's maternal grandfather died at 34 from cancer. Tom is unsure of the site of that cancer, but is aware that of his mother's three siblings, one brother has also been treated for cancer. The genetics nurse in advanced practice explains to Tom that cancer is a term used to describe many diseases that may be unconnected with respect to inherited risk. The diagnoses reported in his family history need to be confirmed before he can be advised concerning his personal cancer risks. The genetics nurse in advanced practice is aware of the genetic basis of cancer and the possibility that the cases of cancer in Tom's family may not be connected, or that the number of cases among his close relatives may be due to a familial cancer syndrome. The nurse asks Tom to obtain written consent from his affected relatives to request relevant details from their medical records, gives Tom a letter for them explaining the reason for the request, and asks him to obtain a copy of his grandfather's death certificate.

The relatives provide consent. In fact his uncle contacts the genetics nurse in advanced practice to ask whether his own children may be at risk. The diagnosis of the deceased grandfather is confirmed as colon cancer on the death certificate, and Tom's mother and uncle are both confirmed to have had colon cancer. However, the pathology reports in both cases indicate the presence of multiple polyps in the colon.

The genetics nurse in advanced practice, after consultation with appropriate cancer specialists, discusses the findings with Tom, explains the genetic basis of the condition, and advises him of the risks to himself and his children. The genetics nurse in advanced practice arranges immediate colonoscopic screening for Tom, as well as offering information for other family members that Tom can share with his family. After a mutation is found in the DNA extracted from a sample of blood from Tom's mother, the genetics nurse in advanced practice discusses similar testing with Tom and other unaffected adult family members. The genetics nurse in advanced practice remains in contact with the family to arrange testing and screening for family members as they reach the appropriate age and to offer psychological support as family members come to terms with their at-risk or affected status. Through correspondence with the family doctor, the genetics nurse in advanced practice provides education to the primary care team about the nature of the condition and the need for colonic surveillance in those who are at risk.

Specialty Certification in Genetics

Certification for genetics nurses is available to nurses practicing in the United States through the Genetic Nursing Credentialing Commission (GNCC) (www.geneticnurse.org) and is evolving worldwide. Although GNCC certification is available to genetics nurses outside the United States, all documents must be submitted in English. Currently this certification is only available to genetics nurses practicing in a clinical setting who spend at least half their time providing genetics-related care. This high practice requirement has limited the number of genetics nurses eligible to apply for certification.

The GNCC began as a subsidiary of ISONG and has evolved into a separate and independent organization. The GNCC supports excellence in genetics nursing practice through the certification of genetics nurses at the basic and advanced practice level. The objective of the GNCC is to enhance the quality of genetics nursing practice through certification of genetics nurses. Certification is based on a professional portfolio of evidence submitted by the nurse (Cook, Kase, Middelton, & Monsen, 2003; Greco & Mahon, 2003). Certification requirements are determined by GNCC and published at www.geneticnurse.org. GNCC offers two credentials: the GCN (Genetics Clinical Nurse) for nurses at the basic practice level and the APNG (Advanced Practice Nurse in Genetics) for nurses at the advanced practice level. Applicants for the GCN must be registered nurses with a baccalaureate in nursing; APNs applying for the APNG must be registered nurses with a master's or doctorate in nursing. Currently GNCC is the only specialty organization in the United States that certifies genetics nurses without a master's in genetics counseling. Nurses with a master's degree in genetics counseling from an accredited program are eligible to apply for genetics counselor certification from the American Board of Genetic Counseling.

The Canadian Association of Genetic Counsellors (CAGC) was established in 1990 and became the credentialing body for genetic counselors in Canada. The CAGC allows nurses without a master's degree in genetics to apply to take the certification examination. Nurses in the United Kingdom can be registered for specialist practice in genetics through a similar system that requires submission of a portfolio to the Registration Board to demonstrate competence (Skirton et al., 2003).

The Future: Genetics and Genomics Knowledge for All Nurses

All licensed registered nurses, regardless of their practice setting, have a role in the delivery of genetics services and the management of genetic information. Nurses require genetics and genomics knowledge to identify, refer, support, and care for persons affected by, or at risk for, manifesting or transmitting conditions or diseases with a genetic component. As the public becomes more aware of the genetic contribution to health and disease, nurses in all areas of practice are being asked to address basic genetics- and genomics-related questions and service needs. A foundation in genetics knowledge is now considered an essential part of baccalaureate nursing education in the United States (AACN, 1998).

Clinically applicable technology and information in the field of human genetics are rapidly expanding and changing healthcare delivery. Nurses in all clinical settings will be increasingly relied on to recognize and appropriately refer clients who can benefit from genetics services. To competently perform these functions, nurses should have a fundamental course in human genetics during their nursing preparation. In addition, didactic content and genetics experience should be integrated into clinical training. Practicing nurses who have not benefited from such instruction should be encouraged to participate in continuing education programs that include basic human genetics concepts, technological applications, and therapeutic modalities applicable to their specific clinical setting.

The core competencies in genetics for all health professionals were defined by the National Coalition for Health Professional Education in Genetics (NCHPEG) in 2001 and updated in 2005. ISONG is represented on the coalition and therefore contributed to the definition of these competencies. These competencies include understanding the basic patterns of inheritance and importance of family history, understanding the role of genetic factors in maintaining health, participating in professional and public education about genetics, and appreciating the sensitivity of genetic information and the need for privacy and confidentiality. The NCHPEG competencies were used by the Genomics Policy Unit in the United Kingdom to define the necessary level of competence required by nurses for professional registration. The validated competency statements were grouped under seven core standards which encapsulate the knowledge, skills, and attitudes required of nurses (Kirk, McDonald, Anstey, & Longley, 2003) . In the United States, essential nursing competencies and curricula guidelines for genetics and genomics have been defined and endorsed both by a consensus panel of nurse experts in September 2005 and also by numerous nursing organizations (Consensus Panel, 2006).

However, it is recognized that few nurses practicing outside specialized genetic settings can claim they are prepared to integrate genetics and genomics into practice. These competencies provide a framework for an education program to prepare nurses to provide genetic clinical service responsibilities.

Genomics offers nurses across the globe the opportunity to apply new technologies to direct patient care. Whether the individual or family has a rare genetic condition, a complex disorder influenced by both genes and environment, an infectious disease for which a gene-based vaccine is developed, or a medical condition requiring individualized pharmacogenomic therapy, it is essential that the nurse understands the biological, ethical, and psychosocial impact of genetics on the care of that person. To expect less is to diminish the professional basis for nursing practice and ultimately to reduce the influence of nursing on outcomes of both health and disease.

Genomics technology is altering the ways in which diseases are prevented, diagnosed, and treated, and will be one of the key drivers of the development of health services in the next decade. Nurses in all healthcare settings and specialties will be expected to help translate these technological developments into effective strategies to benefit clients (Jenkins et al., 2001). Many common diseases, such as cancer, cardiovascular disease, and Alzheimer's disease, previously thought to be the result of lifestyle, dietary, and environmental factors, are now known to have a genetic component. Such diseases are often a result of complex interactions between a person's genetic make-up and a variety of environmental exposures that trigger, accelerate, or exacerbate the disease. This genetic knowledge has increased the complexity of healthcare delivery and resulted in care more tailored to the individual, that must take into account a person's genotype or genetic make-up (Greco, 2003). As longevity continues to increase worldwide, the complexity of genetics nursing practice also increases, because nursing care aimed at the protection, promotion, and optimization of health must evaluate genetic information in the context of advanced biological age, one or more comorbid conditions, and competing health priorities (Greco, 2006).

The modifying influence of particular alleles on the development of complex diseases (such as coronary artery disease, cancer, and diabetes) and the use of genetic testing to identify effective drug therapies are part of this change toward personalized health care. However, nurses are not yet prepared for these innovations (Burton, 2003; Middelton et al., 2002). Genomic era nurses are challenged to develop and implement nursing interventions that take into account a person's genotype, to facilitate the clinical application of genetic technology and to research the impact of genomic information on health outcomes, all within the context of unprecedented information access and global communication (Greco, 2003).

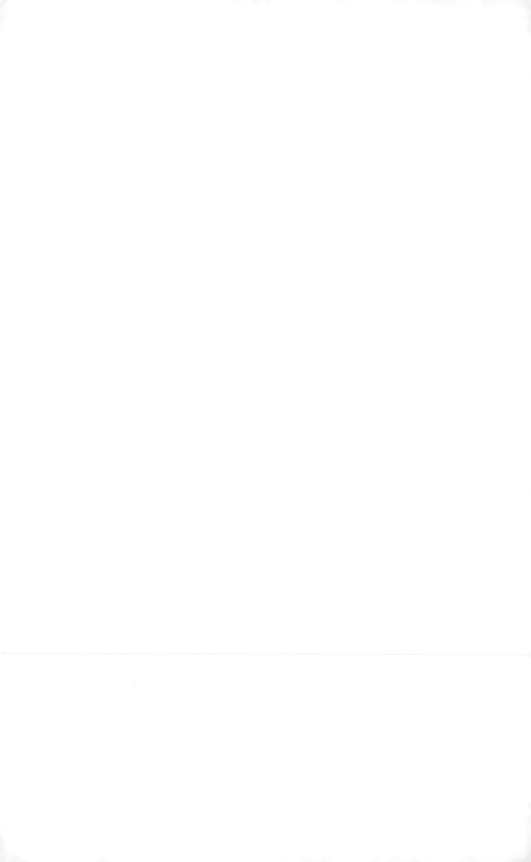

STANDARDS OF GENETICS/GENOMICS NURSING PRACTICE

Standards are authoritative statements in which the nursing profession describes the responsibilities for which nurses are accountable. The document titled *Nursing: Scope and Standards of Practice* (ANA, 2004) is used as a foundation for these genetics specialty scope and standards. This document describes a competent level of professional nursing care and performance for nurses at both the basic and advanced levels of specialty practice. With the exponential growth of knowledge and technological advances in genetics and the evolving role of nurses in this specialty, these standards will be continually evaluated and revised as appropriate.

In this document the word *client* is used broadly to designate the recipient of nursing services, whether it be an individual, family, group, community, or population. Although the wording is often focused on clinical practice, this document is intended to apply to nurses in all areas of genetics nursing practice including, but not limited to, clinical practice, education, research, policy and administration. An example that illustrates this concept follows under assessment: "The genetics nurse collects comprehensive data pertinent to the health of the client or the situation." *Client* here could mean an individual, family, group, community, population, or organization.

In addition, the practice setting lends a context and specificity to who could be a client for genetics nurses. For nurses in education this could be a group of students; for nurses in research this could mean one or more research participants; and for nurses in administration this could mean genetics nurses under their administration. Furthermore:

- For nurses in education it means teaching the collection of comprehensive data pertinent to the health of the client or the situation.

- For nurses in research it applies to the collection of data in the research setting.

- In administration this standard means both assuring that nurses for whom the administrator is responsible collect comprehensive data pertinent to the health of the client or the situation and that institutional policies reflect this standard.

STANDARDS OF PRACTICE

STANDARD 1. ASSESSMENT
The genetics nurse collects comprehensive data pertinent to the client's health or the situation.

Measurement Criteria:

The genetics nurse:

- Collects data in a systematic and ongoing process. Data may include but is not limited to: a three-generation family history, a pedigree constructed using standardized nomenclature, relevant hereditary and nonhereditary risk factors, or physical changes such as dysmorphology associated with a genetic or hereditary disease or condition, etc.

- Bases data collection and assessment on knowledge of human genetic principles, genetics services and resources, current genetics and nursing research, and relevant professional guidelines and recommendations.

- Involves the client, family, other healthcare providers, genetics experts, and the environment, as appropriate in holistic data collection.

- Identifies clients who would benefit from genetics services.

- Prioritizes data collection activities based on the client's condition or anticipated needs or the situation.

- Uses appropriate evidence-based assessment techniques and instruments when possible in collecting pertinent data.

- Uses analytical models and problem-solving tools.

- Documents relevant data in a retrievable format.

- Ensures that data collection, storage, and management are consistent with privacy and confidentiality standards.

Additional Measurement for the Genetics Nurse in Advanced Practice:

The genetics nurse in advanced practice:

- Initiates and interprets screening and diagnostic tests and procedures relevant to the client's current status. These may include, but are not limited to, genetic tests, therapies, and diagnostic procedures.

STANDARD 2. DIAGNOSIS
The genetics nurse analyzes the assessment data to determine diagnoses or issues.

Measurement Criteria:

The genetics nurse:

- Derives the actual and potential diagnoses or issues based on assessment data.

- Validates the diagnoses or issues with the individual, family, community, group, and other health professionals when appropriate and feasible.

- Documents diagnoses, health problems, or issues in a manner that facilitates the determination of the expected outcomes and plan.

Additional Measurement for the Genetics Nurse in Advanced Practice:

The genetics nurse in advanced practice:

- Systematically compares and contrasts clinical findings with normal and abnormal variations and developmental events in formulating a differential diagnosis.

- Utilizes complex data and information obtained during interview, examination, and diagnostic procedures in identifying diagnoses.

- Assists staff in developing and maintaining competency in the diagnostic process.

STANDARD 3. OUTCOMES IDENTIFICATION
The genetics nurse identifies expected outcomes for a plan individualized to the client or the situation.

Measurement Criteria:

The genetics nurse:

- Involves the individual, family, community, or group and other healthcare and genetics providers in formulating the expected outcomes when possible and appropriate.

- Derives culturally appropriate expected outcomes from the diagnoses.

- Considers associated risks, benefits, costs, current scientific evidence, and genetic information when formulating expected outcomes.

- Defines expected outcomes in terms of the client, client values, ethical considerations, culture, environment, or situation.

- Includes a time estimate for attainment of expected outcomes.

- Develops expected outcomes that provide direction for continuity of care.

- Modifies expected outcomes based on changes in the status of the client or re-evaluation of the situation.

- Derives expected outcomes that reflect current scientific knowledge in clinical application of human genetics research and technology, and use of genetics resources.

- Documents expected outcomes as measurable goals when possible.

Additional Measurement for the Genetics Nurse in Advanced Practice:

The genetics nurse in advanced practice:

- Identifies expected outcomes that incorporate scientific evidence and are achievable through implementation of evidence-based principles.

- Identifies expected outcomes that incorporate cost and clinical effectiveness, client satisfaction, and continuity and consistency among healthcare providers and genetics services.

- Supports the use of clinical guidelines linked to positive client outcomes.

STANDARD 4. PLANNING
The genetics nurse develops a plan that prescribes strategies and alternatives to attain expected outcomes.

Measurement Criteria:

The genetics nurse:

- Develops an individualized plan considering the characteristics or situation of the client, family, community, or group (e.g., age, genetic status, genetic risk, culture).

- Develops the plan in conjunction with the client, family, group, healthcare team members and genetics experts, and others as appropriate.

- Includes strategies within the plan that address each of the identified diagnoses or issues, including genetics-related diagnoses or issues. These strategies may include, but are not limited to, strategies for promotion and restoration of health, prevention of illness, injury, and disease, and facilitating maximum wellness.

- Provides for continuity of care within the plan.

- Incorporates an implementation pathway or timeline within the plan.

- Establishes the plan priorities with the client, family, and others as appropriate.

- Uses the plan to provide direction to other members of the healthcare team.

- Defines the plan to reflect current statutes, rules, regulations, and standards.

- Integrates current scientific evidence, trends, and research affecting care in the planning process.

- Documents the plan of care in a manner that uses standardized language or recognized terminology.

- Considers the economic impact of the plan.

Continued ▶

Additional Measurement for the Genetics Nurse in Advanced Practice:

The genetics nurse in advanced practice:

- Identifies assessment, diagnostic, surveillance, and management strategies, therapeutic interventions, and risk-reduction plans that reflect current evidence and expert clinical knowledge.

- Selects or designs strategies to meet the multifaceted needs of complex clients.

- Includes the synthesis of clients' values and beliefs regarding nursing and medical therapies within the plan.

STANDARD 5. IMPLEMENTATION
The genetics nurse implements the identified plan.

Measurement Criteria:

The genetics nurse:

- Implements the plan in a safe, timely, and appropriate manner.
- Documents implementation and any modifications, including changes to or omissions from the identified plan.
- Uses evidence-based interventions and treatments unique to the client's needs.
- Uses healthcare, community, and genetics resources and systems to implement the plan.
- Collaborates with nursing colleagues, genetics experts, and others as appropriate to implement the plan.
- Implements the plan using principles and concepts of project or systems management when appropriate.
- Fosters organizational systems that support implementation of the plan.

Additional Measurement for the Genetics Nurse in Advanced Practice:

The genetics nurse in advanced practice:

- Facilitates utilization of systems, community, and genetics resources to implement the plan.
- Supports collaboration with nursing colleagues, genetics professionals, other disciplines, and others as appropriate to implement the plan.
- Incorporates new knowledge and strategies to initiate change in nursing care practices if it would improve desired outcomes or if desired outcomes are not achieved.

STANDARD 5A. COORDINATION OF CARE

The genetics nurse coordinates care delivery for, but is not limited to, clients with genetic conditions, genetic predisposition, or complex diseases with a genetic component.

Measurement Criteria:

The genetics nurse:

- Coordinates implementation of the plan.

- Documents the coordination of care according to appropriate guidelines and addressing privacy and confidentiality.

- Provides coordination of services with consideration of the client's informed choice and right to privacy, confidentiality, and nondiscrimination.

- Identifies available genetic support groups or networking services when appropriate.

Additional Measurement for the Genetics Nurse in Advanced Practice:

The genetics nurse in advanced practice:

- Provides leadership in the coordination of multidisciplinary health care for integrated delivery of client care services. This includes, but is not limited to, coordination of genetics services or programs.

- Provides leadership in the coordination of genetics research and genetics education when appropriate.

- Synthesizes data and information to prescribe necessary system and community support measures, including environmental modifications.

- Coordinates system, community, and genetics resources that enhance delivery of care.

STANDARD 5B. HEALTH TEACHING AND HEALTH PROMOTION
The genetics nurse employs strategies to promote health and a safe environment.

Measurement Criteria:

The genetics nurse:

- Provides health teaching that addresses such topics as healthy lifestyles, risk-reducing behaviors, developmental needs, activities of daily living, preventive self-care, management of health risk associated with genetic risk factors, and management of genetic conditions.

- Uses health promotion and health teaching methods appropriate to the client's developmental level, learning needs, readiness, ability to learn, language preference, and culture.

- Seeks opportunities for feedback and evaluation of the effectiveness of the health teaching and health promotion strategies used.

- Uses genetics education and other strategies to promote health and safe environments and to minimize the potential effects of genetic alterations associated with disease risk.

- Provides genetics education that includes information on risk assessment, risk reduction, health promotion, and disease prevention strategies appropriate for persons at risk for or carrying a disease-associated genetic alteration.

Additional Measurement for the Genetics Nurse in Advanced Practice:

The genetics nurse in advanced practice:

- Synthesizes scientific and empirical evidence on learning theories, behavioral change theories, epidemiology, and other relevant theories and frameworks when designing health information and client education.

- Synthesizes scientific and empirical evidence on risk assessment, risk behaviors, risk reduction, surveillance and management of high risk populations, and other relevant information when designing health information and client education.

Continued ▶

Standards of Genetics Nursing Practice

- Designs health information, client education, and health promotion plans appropriate to the developmental level, learning needs, readiness to learn, and cultural values and beliefs of the target audience.

- Evaluates genetics health information resources (e.g., Internet, media, professional and lay publications) for accuracy, readability, and comprehensibility to help clients, families, groups, or communities access quality health information.

- Develops health promotion, surveillance, management, and risk-reduction plans that promote healthy behaviors and optimum wellness for individuals, families, groups, or communities at risk for, diagnosed with, or affected by genetic or hereditary diseases and conditions.

STANDARD 5C. CONSULTATION
The genetics nurse provides consultation to influence the identified plan of care, enhance the abilities of others, and effect change.

Measurement Criteria:

The genetics nurse:

- Synthesizes clinical data, theoretical frameworks, and evidence when providing consultation.

- Facilitates the effectiveness of a consultation by involving the client in decision-making and negotiating role responsibilities.

- Communicates consultation recommendations that facilitate change.

- Promotes awareness and discussion of ethical dimensions such as privacy, confidentiality, informed consent, truth telling, disclosure, and nondiscrimination during the consultation process.

Additional Measurement for the Genetics Nurse in Advanced Practice:

The genetics nurse in advanced practice:

- Synthesizes data, information, theoretical frameworks, and evidence when providing consultation.

- Facilitates the effectiveness of a consultation by involving the stakeholders in the decision-making process.

- Communicates consultation recommendations that influence the identified plan, facilitate understanding by involved stakeholders, enhance the work of others, and effect change.

- Engages in consultation activities related to genetic health issues.

STANDARD 5D. PRESCRIPTIVE AUTHORITY AND TREATMENT

The genetics nurse in advanced practice uses prescriptive authority, procedures, referrals, treatments, and therapies in accordance with the applicable national, regional, or local laws and regulations.

Measurement for the Genetics Nurse in Advanced Practice:

The genetics nurse in advanced practice:

- Prescribes evidence-based treatments, therapies, and procedures considering the client's comprehensive healthcare needs.

- Prescribes pharmacologic agents based on a current knowledge of pharmacology, physiology, and pharmacogenomics.

- Prescribes specific pharmacological agents and treatments based on clinical indicators, risk assessment, the client's status and needs, and results of diagnostic and laboratory tests, including genetic tests.

- Evaluates therapeutic and potential adverse effects of pharmacological and non-pharmacological treatments, including appropriate genetic therapies.

- Provides individuals and families with information about intended effects and potential adverse effects of proposed prescriptive therapies, including the potential impact of genetic alterations on drug response.

- Provides information about costs, and alternative treatments and procedures, as appropriate.

STANDARD 5E. COUNSELING

The genetics nurse uses counseling interventions to assist clients in understanding, adapting to, and using genetic information.

Measurement Criteria:

The genetics nurse:

- Uses active listening and therapeutic communication skills.
- Provides counseling that is anticipatory, therapeutic, facilitative, supportive, and sensitive.
- Provides counseling that is culturally sensitive, is consistent with the client's values and preferences, promotes informed decision-making, and is based on mutually agreed-upon goals.
- Documents counseling interventions in a retrievable format in a way that protects client confidentiality and privacy.
- Respects client autonomy when counseling.
- Provides counseling in a nonjudgmental environment where relevant concerns and emotions can be expressed.
- Provides an environment in which the emotional and psychological impact of the genetic condition or risk can be explored safely.

Additional Measurement for the Genetics Nurse in Advanced Practice:

The genetics nurse in advanced practice:

- Provides genetic counseling and education specific to genetic and genomic issues relevant to care. (Genetic counseling, for example, might include discussing the potential benefits and limitations of genetic testing for disease-associated mutations, alternatives to genetic testing, and the implications of potential genetic test results.)
- Integrates current scientific evidence, trends, and research affecting care in the genetic counseling process.

STANDARD 6. EVALUATION
The genetics nurse evaluates progress toward attainment of desired outcomes.

Measurement Criteria:

The genetics nurse:

- Conducts a systematic, ongoing, and criterion-based evaluation of the outcomes in relation to the prescribed plan and proposed timeline.

- Includes the client, family, team members, genetics experts, and others as appropriate in the evaluation process.

- Evaluates effectiveness of the planned strategies in relation to client responses and the attainment of expected outcomes.

- Documents the results of the evaluation and any revisions in a systematic and standardized format.

- Uses ongoing assessment data to revise diagnoses, outcomes, plan of care, and implementation as needed.

- Disseminates the results to the client and others involved in the care or situation, as appropriate in accordance with appropriate standards of practice, laws or regulations, and ethical standards.

- Reflects awareness of and sensitivity to ethical, legal, and social issues in the evaluation process.

Additional Measurement for the Genetics Nurse in Advanced Practice:

The genetics nurse in advanced practice:

- Evaluates the accuracy of the diagnosis and effectiveness of the interventions in relationship to the client's attainment of expected outcomes.

- Synthesizes the results of the evaluation analyses to determine the impact of the plan on the affected individuals, families, groups, communities, institutions, networks, and organizations. In research involving human subjects this includes research participants.

- Uses the results of the evaluation analyses to make or recommend process or structural changes, including policy, procedure, or protocol documentation, as appropriate.

Standards of Professional Performance

Standard 7. Quality of Practice
The genetics nurse systematically enhances the quality and effectiveness of genetics nursing practice.

Measurement Criteria:

The genetics nurse:

- Demonstrates quality by documenting the application of the nursing process in a responsible, accountable, and ethical manner.
- Uses results from quality improvement activities to initiate changes in nursing practice and in the healthcare delivery system. This includes, but is not limited to, genetics nursing practice and the delivery of genetics services, as appropriate.
- Uses creativity and innovation in nursing practice to improve care delivery.
- Incorporates new knowledge to initiate changes in nursing practice when appropriate or if desired outcomes are not achieved.
- Participates in quality improvement activities as appropriate. Such activities may include but are not limited to:
  - Identifying aspects of practice important for monitoring,
  - Using relevant indicators to monitor quality and effectiveness of nursing practice,
  - Collecting data to monitor quality and effectiveness of nursing practice,
  - Analyzing quality data to identify opportunities for improving nursing practice,
  - Formulating recommendations to improve nursing practice and client outcomes,
  - Implementing activities to enhance the quality of nursing practice,
  - Developing, implementing, and evaluating policies, procedures, and guidelines to improve the quality of practice,

Continued ▶

- Participating in interdisciplinary, multidisciplinary, or transdisciplinary teams to evaluate clinical care or genetics or health services,

- Participating in efforts to minimize costs and unnecessary duplication,

- Analyzing factors related to safety, satisfaction, effectiveness, and cost–benefit outcomes,

- Analyzing organizational systems for barriers,

- Implementing processes to remove or decrease barriers within organizational systems, and

- Documenting results of quality assessment and improvement activities.

- Strives to obtain and maintain professional certification or credentialing, if available, in their area of expertise.

Additional Measurement for the Genetics Nurse in Advanced Practice:

The genetics nurse in advanced practice:

- Designs quality improvement initiatives.

- Implements initiatives to evaluate the need for change.

- Evaluates the practice environment in relation to existing evidence, identifying opportunities for the generation and use of research.

- Strives to obtain and maintain professional certification or credentialing as an advanced practice nurse, if available, in their area of expertise.

- Evaluates the quality of nursing care rendered in relation to existing evidence, identifying opportunities for the generation and use of research.

STANDARD 8. EDUCATION
The genetics nurse attains knowledge and competency that reflects current nursing practice.

Measurement Criteria:

The genetics nurse:

- Participates in educational activities related to appropriate knowledge bases and professional issues.

- Demonstrates a commitment to lifelong learning through self-reflection and inquiry to identify learning needs.

- Seeks experiences and learning opportunities that reflect current practice in order to maintain skills and competence in clinical practice or role performance.

- Acquires knowledge and skills appropriate to the genetics specialty, practice setting, role, or situation.

- Maintains professional records that provide evidence of competency and lifelong learning.

- Seeks experiences and formal and independent learning activities to maintain and develop clinical and professional skills and knowledge.

- Attains core competencies in genetics for all nurses as outlined by appropriate national or international published professional guidelines and recommendations. An example of such competencies are those in the most current version of *Essential Nursing Competencies and Curricula Guidelines for Genetics and Genomics* (Consensus Panel 2006).

- Participates in efforts to educate all nurses and other healthcare providers regarding fundamental knowledge and competencies in genetics related to nursing practice.

- Helps educate nurses and other healthcare providers in translating genetics information and technology into effective strategies to benefit individuals, families, communities, and groups.

Additional Measurement for the Genetics Nurse in Advanced Practice:

The genetics nurse in advanced practice:

- Uses current healthcare research findings and other evidence to expand knowledge, enhance role performance, and increase knowledge of professional issues.

Standards of Professional Performance

STANDARD 9. PROFESSIONAL PRACTICE EVALUATION

The genetics nurse evaluates one's own nursing practice in relationship to professional practice standards and guidelines, relevant statutes, rules, and regulations.

Measurement Criteria:

The genetics nurse:

- Provides age-appropriate care in a culturally and ethnically sensitive manner.

- Engages regularly in self-evaluation of practice and role performance to identify areas of competence and areas of developmental need, especially related to genetics nursing practice.

- Obtains informal feedback regarding one's own practice from clients, peers, professional colleagues, and others.

- Engages in a formal process seeking feedback regarding role performance.

- Participates in systematic peer review as appropriate.

- Takes action to achieve goals identified during the evaluation process.

- Provides rationales for practice beliefs, decisions, and actions as part of the informal and formal evaluation processes.

Additional Measurement for the Genetics Nurse in Advanced Practice:

The genetics nurse in advanced practice:

- Engages in a formal process seeking feedback regarding one's own practice from clients, peers, professional colleagues, and others.

STANDARD 10. COLLEGIALITY
The genetics nurse interacts with and contributes to the professional development of peers and colleagues.

Measurement Criteria:

The genetics nurse:

- Shares knowledge and skills with peers and colleagues as evidenced by activities such as client care conferences, formal and informal presentations, publications, and other practice opportunities.

- Provides peers with feedback regarding their practice and role performance.

- Interacts with peers and colleagues to enhance one's own professional nursing practice and role performance.

- Maintains compassionate and caring relationships with peers and colleagues.

- Uses appropriate strategies to promote and maintain professional commitment towards self, clients, and other healthcare professionals.

- Supports and facilitates professional development of peers and colleagues regarding genetics knowledge, genetics competencies, and the application of genetics information and technology to client care.

Additional Measurement for the Genetics Nurse in Advanced Practice:

The genetics nurse in advanced practice:

- Mentors other nurses, professional colleagues, students, and others as appropriate.

- Models expert practice to team members, professional colleagues, genetics experts, healthcare consumers, and others.

- Participates in multidisciplinary, interdisciplinary, and transdisciplinary teams that contribute to role development and, directly or indirectly, advance nursing practice and health services.

STANDARD 11. COLLABORATION
The genetics nurse collaborates with the client, family, and others in the conduct of nursing practice.

Measurement Criteria:

The genetics nurse:

- Communicates with clients, families, communities, groups, health-care providers, genetics experts, and others as appropriate regarding client care and the nurse's role in the provision of that care.

- Collaborates in creating a documented plan, focused on outcomes and decisions related to care and delivery of services, that indicates communication with clients, families, healthcare providers, genetics experts, and others as appropriate.

- Partners with others to effect change and generate positive outcomes through knowledge of the client or situation.

- Documents referrals, including provisions for continuity of care.

- Practices as an effective team member in a multidisciplinary, inter-disciplinary, or transdisciplinary team.

- Partners with others to enhance health care and, ultimately, client care through team activities such as education, consultation, management, technological development, and research opportunities.

- Documents plans, communications, rationale for plan changes, and collaborative discussions.

Additional Measurement for the Genetics Nurse in Advanced Practice:

The genetics nurse in advanced practice:

- Partners with others to enhance client care through multi-disciplinary, interdisciplinary, or transdisciplinary team activities such as education, consultation, management, technological development, and research opportunities.

- Facilitates a multidisciplinary, interdisciplinary, or transdisciplinary team process with other members of the healthcare team.

- Practices in a leadership role in multidisciplinary, interdisciplinary, and transdisciplinary teams in the specialty role.

Standard 12. Ethics

The genetics nurse employs ethical provisions in all areas of practice.

Measurement Criteria:

The genetics nurse:

- Is guided by a code of ethics for nurses such as *Code of Ethics for Nurses with Interpretive Statements* (ANA, 2001), *ICN Code of Ethics for Nurses* (ICN, 2001), or a relevant national code of ethics.

- Provides care and services in a manner that preserves and protects the client's autonomy, dignity, and rights.

- Maintains client confidentiality within legal and regulatory parameters.

- Serves as a client advocate assisting clients in developing skills for self-advocacy.

- Maintains a therapeutic and professional client–nurse relationship within appropriate professional role boundaries. This includes, but is not limited to, faculty–student, researcher–participant, and supervisor–subordinate relationships.

- Demonstrates a commitment to practicing self-care, managing stress, and connecting with self and others.

- Contributes to resolving ethical issues of clients, colleagues, or systems as evidenced in such activities as participating on ethics committees.

- Identifies ethical dilemmas in clinical practice and uses resources in formulating ethical responses.

- Addresses ethical issues related to genetics information.

- Participates in formulating guidelines about the ethical considerations of new and existing genetics services and technology.

- Reports illegal, incompetent, or impaired practices.

- Participates on multidisciplinary and interdisciplinary teams that address ethical risks, benefits, and outcomes.

- Informs administrators or others of the risks, benefits, and outcomes of programs and decisions that affect healthcare delivery.

Continued ▶

Additional Measurement for the Genetics Nurse in Advanced Practice:

The genetics nurse in advanced practice:

- Informs the client of the risks, benefits, and outcomes of healthcare regimes such as genetic testing.

- Addresses ethical issues related to the provision of genetic counseling services, such as informed consent, confidentiality, autonomy, and beneficence.

- Participates in efforts to address ethical issues such as ethics committees and institutional review boards (IRBs).

STANDARD 13. RESEARCH
The genetics nurse integrates research findings into practice.

Measurement Criteria:

The genetics nurse:

- Uses the best available evidence, including research findings, to guide practice decisions.
- Actively participates in research activities at various levels appropriate to the nurse's position, education, and practice environment. Such activities may include but are not limited to:
  - Applying research findings to genetics nursing practice and assisting others to do so,
  - Consulting with research experts and colleagues as necessary,
  - Critiquing research for application to genetics nursing practice,
  - Developing, conducting, or evaluating genetics nursing research,
  - Identifying clinical problems suitable for genetics nursing research,
  - Participating In hospital-, organization-, or community-based research committees or programs,
  - Participating in multidisciplinary genetics research,
  - Participating in human subject protection activities as appropriate,
  - Participating in data collection (surveys, pilot projects, formal studies),
  - Sharing research activities and findings with peers and others,
  - Critically analyzing and interpreting research for application to practice,
  - Using research findings in the development of policies, procedures, guidelines, and standards of practice in client care,
  - Incorporating research as a basis for learning, and
  - Participating in cross-disciplinary research with other health professionals, genetics experts, and others.

Continued ▶

Additional Measurement for the Genetics Nurse in Advanced Practice:

The genetics nurse in advanced practice:

- Contributes to nursing knowledge by conducting or synthesizing research that discovers, examines, and evaluates knowledge, theories, criteria, and creative approaches to improve healthcare and nursing practice.

- Contributes to nursing science, genetics science, and related sciences by conducting or synthesizing research.

- Formally disseminates research findings through activities such as presentations at professional conferences and meetings, peer-reviewed and other publications, consultation, and journal clubs.

Standard 14. Resource Utilization

The genetics nurse considers factors related to safety, effectiveness, cost, and impact on practice in the planning and delivery of nursing services.

Measurement Criteria:

The genetics nurse:

- Evaluates factors such as safety, efficacy, availability, cost, benefits, and efficiencies when choosing practice options that would result in equivalent outcomes.

- Assists the client (and family if appropriate) in identifying and securing available, appropriate services to address health-related needs.

- Assigns or delegates tasks based on the needs and condition of the client, potential for harm, stability of the client's condition, complexity of the task, and predictability of the outcome.

- Assists the client and family in becoming informed consumers about the options, costs, risks, and benefits of treatment and care.

- Develops innovative solutions and applies strategies to obtain appropriate resources.

- Secures organizational resources to ensure a work environment conducive to completing the identified plan and outcomes.

- Develops evaluation methods to measure safety and effectiveness for interventions and outcomes.

- Promotes activities that assist others, as appropriate, in becoming informed about costs, risks, and benefits of care, or of the plan and solution.

- Participates in ongoing resource utilization review.

Additional Measurement for the Genetics Nurse in Advanced Practice:

The genetics nurse in advanced practice:

- Uses organizational and community resources to formulate multidisciplinary, interdisciplinary, or transdisciplinary plans of care.

Continued ▶

- Develops innovative solutions for client care problems that address effective resource utilization and maintenance of quality.

- Develops evaluation strategies to demonstrate cost-effectiveness, cost-benefit, and efficiency factors associated with nursing practice.

STANDARD 15. LEADERSHIP
The genetics nurse provides leadership in the professional practice setting and the profession.

Measurement Criteria:

The genetics nurse:

- Engages in teamwork as a team player and a team builder.

- Works to create and maintain healthy environments in local, regional, national, or international communities.

- Displays the ability to define a clear vision, the associated goals, and a plan to implement and measure progress.

- Demonstrates a commitment to continuous, lifelong learning for self and others.

- Teaches others to succeed by mentoring and other strategies.

- Exhibits creativity and flexibility through times of change.

- Demonstrates energy, excitement, and a passion for quality work.

- Willingly accepts unintentional mistakes by self and others.

- Creates a culture in which risk taking is not only safe, but expected, when reasonable benefits are anticipated.

- Inspires loyalty through valuing of people as the most precious asset in an organization.

- Directs the coordination of care across settings and among caregivers, including oversight of licensed and unlicensed personnel in any assigned or delegated tasks.

- Serves in key roles in the work setting by participating on committees, councils, and administrative teams.

- Promotes the advancement of the profession through involvement with professional organizations.

- Promotes advancement of genetics nursing through participation in professional and community organizations.

- Works to influence decision-making bodies to improve client care, healthcare services, and policies.

Continued ▶

- Promotes communication of information and advancement of the profession through writing, publishing, and presentations for professional or lay audiences.

Additional Measurement for the Genetics Nurse in Advanced Practice:

The genetics nurse in advanced practice:

- Works to influence decision-making bodies to improve client care, health services, and health-related policies at the local, community, national, and international level.
- Provides leadership and direction to enhance the effectiveness of the healthcare team.
- Initiates and revises protocols or guidelines to reflect evidence-based practice, to reflect accepted changes in care management, or to address emerging problems.
- Promotes communication of information and improvement of advanced nursing practice through writing, publishing, and presentations for professional or lay audiences.
- Serves in leadership roles in professional and community organizations at the local, community, national, and international level.

REFERENCES

All URLs were accessed on August 28, 2006.

American Association of Colleges of Nursing (AACN). (1998). *The essentials of baccalaureate education for professional nursing practice.* Washington, DC: AACN.

American Nurses Association (ANA). (2001). *Code of ethics for nurses with interpretive statements.* Washington, DC: Nursesbooks.org.

American Nurses Association. (2003). *Nursing's social policy statement.* Washington, DC: Nursesbooks.org.

American Nurses Association. (2004). *Nursing: Scope and standards of practice.* Washington, DC: Nursesbooks.org.

Ando, H. (2001). *Towards the practice of genetic nursing based on regional characteristics.* Abstract presented at the annual conference of the International Society of Nurses in Genetics, San Diego, CA.

Ando, H., Takeda, Y., & Williams. (2001) *Ethical issues in genetic nursing platform presentations.* December. Japan Academy of Nursing Science, Kobe.

Arimori, N., Nakagomi, S., Mizoguchi, M., Nakagomi, S., Ando, H., Morita, M., Mori, A., & Horiuchi, S. (2000). *The core competence of genetic nursing in Japan.* Abstract presented at the International Society of Nursing in Genetics Conference, Philadelphia, PA.

Burton, H. (2003). *Addressing genetics: Delivering health. A strategy for advancing the dissemination and application of genetics knowledge throughout our health professions.* Cambridge: Cambridge Genetics Knowledge Park.

Consensus Panel on Genetic/Genomic Nursing Competencies (2006). *Essential nursing competencies and curricula guidelines for genetics and genomics*, Silver Spring, MD: Nursesbooks.org. Also available online at http://www.genome.gov or http://www.nursingworld.org/ethics/genetics/competencies.htm.

Cook, S. S., Kase, R., Middelton, L., & Monsen, R. B. (2003). Portfolio evaluation for professional competence: Credentialing in genetics for nurses. *Journal of Professional Nursing, 19*(2), 85–90.

Department of Health. (2003). *Our inheritance, our future. Realizing the potential of genetics in the NHS*. http://www.dh.gov.uk/assetRoot/04/01/92/39/04019239.pdf.

Education Working Group of the Association of Genetic Nurses and Counsellors. (2001). The registration of genetic counsellors. www.agnc.org.uk/Registration/registration.htm.

Forsman, I. (1994). Evolution of the nursing role in genetics. *Journal of Obstetric, Gynecologic, and Neonatal Nursing, 23*(6), 481–486.

Greco, K. E. (2003). Nursing in the genomic era: Nurturing our genetic nature. *MEDSURG Nursing, 12*(5), 307–312.

Greco, K. E. (2006) Cancer screening in older adults in an era of genomics and longevity. *Seminars in Oncology Nursing, 22*(1), 10–19.

Greco, K. E., & Mahon, S. M. (2003). Genetics nursing practice enters a new era with credentialing. *Internet Journal of Advanced Nursing Practice, 5*(2).

Guttmacher, A. E., Collins, F. S., & Drazen, J. M. (2004). *Genomic Medicine*. Baltimore: John Hopkins University Press.

International Council of Nurses (2001). *The ICN Code of Ethics for Nurses*. http://www.icn.ch/icncode.pdf.

International Society of Nurses in Genetics (ISONG) & American Nurses Association (ANA). (1998). *Statement on the scope and standards of genetics clinical nursing practice.* Washington, DC: American Nurses Publishing.

Jenkins, J. F., Prows, C., Dimond, E., Monsen, R., & Williams, J. (2001). Recommendations for educating nurses in genetics. *Journal of Professional Nursing 17*(6), 283–290.

Kirk, M., McDonald, K., Anstey, S., & Longley, M. (2003). *Fit for practice in the genetics era: A competence-based education framework for nurses, midwives and health visitors.* University of Glamoran, Wales: National Health Services Genetics Team. http://www.glam.ac.uk/socsschool/research/gpu/FinalReport.pdf.

Lashley, F. (1997). Nursing and genetics: The past and the future. In F. Lashley (Ed.) *The genetics revolution: Implications for nursing .* Washington, DC: American Academy of Nursing.

Middelton, L., Dimond, E., Calzone, K., Davis, J. & Jenkins, J. (2002). The role of the nurse in cancer genetics. *Cancer Nursing 25*(3), 196–206.

Mizoguchi, M., Arimori, N., Nakogomi, S., Morita, M., Ando, H., Akiko, M., & Horiuchi, S. (2002). *Evaluation of a pilot program in genetic nursing for general nurses in Japan.* Abstract presented at the annual conference (October) of the International Society of Nurses in Genetics, Baltimore, MD.

Mizoguchi, M. (2004). *Delivery of genetic services in Japan: How nurses are involved.* Abstract presented at the annual conference (October) at the International Society of Nurses in Genetics, Toronto, Canada.

Monsen, R. B. (Ed.) (2005). *Genetics nursing portfolios: A new model for credentialing.* Silver Spring, MD: Nursesbooks.org.

Morita, M., Ando, H., Mizoguchi, M., Arimori, N., Nakagomi, S., Mori, A., & Horiuchi, S. (2003). *Implementation and evaluation of a genetic nursing program for the general nurse in Japan.* Abstract presented at the annual conference (November) at the International Society of Nurses in Genetics, Los Angeles, CA.

National Coalition for Health Professions Education in Genetics (NCHPEG) (2005). *Core competencies in genetics essential for all health care professionals.* http://www.nchpeg.org/.

Skirton, H., Barnes, C., Curtis, G., & Walford-Moore, J. (1997). The role and practice of the genetic nurse: Report of the AGNC working party. *Journal of Medical Genetics 34,* 141–7.

Skirton, H., Barnes, C., Guilbert, P., Kershaw, A., Kerzin-Storrar, L., Patch, C., Curtis, G., & Walford-Moore, J. (1998). Recommendations for education and training of genetic nurses and counsellors in the United Kingdom. *Journal of Medical Genetics 35*(5), 410–412.

Skirton, H., Kerzin-Storrar, L., Patch, C., Barnes, C., Guilbert, P., Dolling, C., Kershaw, A., Baines, E., & Stirling, D. (2003). Genetic counsellors: A registration system to assure competence in practice in the United Kingdom. *Community Genetics 6*(3), 182–183.

GLOSSARY

Advanced Practice Nurse in Genetics (APNG). A nurse who holds an APNG Credential from the Genetic Nursing Credentialing Commission (www.geneticnurse.org). A registered nurse with at least a master's degree in nursing who has achieved genetic expertise through formal genetic education, continuing education, and clinical experience.

Allele. One of the multiple forms of a gene at a particular locus that can occur within a population. The wild type allele is the most common form of a gene found within a population. Alternative forms of the wild type allele are typically designated by letters and numbers that refer to the type and location of a variation within the DNA sequence of a gene or its regulatory elements.

Assessment. The process by which a registered nurse, through interaction with the client and other healthcare providers, collects and analyzes data. Assessment may include the following dimensions: physical, psychological, sociocultural, spiritual, cognitive, functional abilities, developmental, economic, and lifestyle.

Caregiver. A person who provides direct care for another, such as a child, dependent adult, the disabled, or the chronically ill.

Client. A recipient of nursing services, whether an individual, a family, a community, or a population. When the client is an individual, the focus is on the health state and actual or potential problems or needs of the individual. When the client is a family or group, the focus is on the health or genetic susceptibilities of the unit as a whole or the reciprocal effects of the individual's health state on the other members of the unit. When the client is a community or population, the focus is on personal and environmental health and genetic risk factors that influence health of the community or population. Examples include:

- A person or a couple who has or is at risk for having a child with a hereditary or genetic condition or congenital anomaly
- An asymptomatic person or family with a genetic susceptibility for developing a disorder or disease
- A person or group who needs or requests genetic information

- A group, community, or population with or at risk for hereditary or genetic conditions

In the education setting the client includes the students being taught, and in research the client includes participants in the research setting.

Code of ethics. A statement of the primary goals, values, and obligations of a profession.

Congenital anomaly. An abnormality of structure or form present at birth that may or may not be inherited or genetic. *Birth defect*, a common synonym for congenital anomaly, is sometimes considered offensive.

Continuity of care. An interdisciplinary process facilitates the client's transition between settings and healthcare providers, based on changing needs and available resources. This process includes patients, families, and significant others in the development of a coordinated plan of care.

Credentialing in genetics nursing. The process of documenting a nurse's clinical competency in genetics nursing based on reviewing a professional portfolio of accomplishments submitted by the nurse. Credentialing requirements determined by the Genetic Nursing Credentialing Commission (GNCC) are published at www.geneticnurse.org. GNCC offers two credentials: the GCN (Genetics Clinical Nurse) for nurses at the basic practice level and the APNG (Advanced Practice Nurse in Genetics) for nurses at the advanced practice level.

Criteria. Relevant, measurable indicators of the standards of practice and professional performance.

Diagnosis. A clinical judgment about the client's response to actual or potential health conditions or needs. The diagnosis is the basis for the plan to achieve expected outcomes. Registered nurses utilize nursing and medical diagnoses depending upon educational and clinical preparation and legal authority.

Dysmorphology. The study of prenatal abnormal structural development. These can include major and minor congenital anomalies. Major anomalies require medical, surgical, or developmental intervention; minor anomalies do not.

Dysmorphology assessment. A physical examination that specifically assesses the presence of major and minor anomalies to determine a pattern consistent with a genetic condition.

Evaluation. The process of determining both the client's progress toward attainment of expected outcomes and the effectiveness of nursing care.

Evidence-based. Founded on the best available evidence, moderated by patient circumstances and preferences, and applied to improve the quality of clinical judgments derived from clinical research.

Expected outcomes. End results that are measurable, desirable, and observable, and translate into observable behaviors

Family. Biologic and social relationships identified by the client as family.

Gene. The basic physical and functional unit of heredity. A gene is encoded by a linear sequence of bases at a specific location within a DNA strand; it controls the formation of proteins or regulates other genes.

Genetic condition. An anomaly, behavior, disease, issue, or predisposition caused or influenced by genes which may affect one's health or abilities and may or may not be inherited. A **hereditary condition** is one type of genetic condition.

Genetic predisposition. Increased susceptibility to a particular disease due to the presence of one or more gene mutations that is associated with an increased risk for the disease, and/or a family history that indicates an increased risk for the disease, which may or may not result in actual development of the disease.

Genetic testing. Examination of blood, body fluids, or body tissues for biochemical, chromosome, and DNA or RNA variations to determine the presence of a disease or disorder or the predisposition for disease. Outside the realm of disease, genetic testing (DNA/RNA) is also being used for pharmacogenomics, paternity identification, and forensics.

Genetics. The study of individual genes and their impact on single-gene disorders.

Genetics Clinical Nurse (GCN). A nurse who holds a GCN Credential from the Genetic Nursing Credentialing Commission (www.geneticnurse.org). A registered nurse with a bachelor's degree in nursing who has achieved genetic expertise through formal genetic education, continuing education, and clinical experience.

Genetics counseling. An exchange of information between genetics healthcare professionals and clients. The genetics healthcare professional seeks to impartially and completely provide comprehensive information regarding the medical facts of, and expectations for, the course of the disorder and its expected course, mode of inheritance, recurrence risks, and diagnostic and treatment options, to promote adjustment and to support the chosen course of action.

Genetics/genomics nursing. The protection, promotion, and optimization of health and abilities, prevention of illness and injury, and alleviation of suffering through the diagnosis of human response and advocacy in the care of the genetic and genomic health of individuals, families, communities, and populations. This includes health issues, genetic conditions, and diseases or susceptibilities to diseases that are caused or influenced by genes in interaction with other risk factors that may require nursing care.

Genetics nursing practice. Providing client-centered nursing care, education, or research based on understanding the underlying genomics of individuals, families, communities, or populations affected by, or at risk for, a disease or condition with a genetic component.

Genomics. The study of all the genes in the human genome together or as a subset, including their interactions with each other, the environment, and the influence of other psychosocial and cultural factors.

Health. An experience that is often expressed in terms of wellness and illness, and may occur in the presence or absence of disease or injury.

Hereditary condition. A condition caused or significantly influenced by an allele or pair of alleles that is passed to subsequent generations through the egg or sperm.

Implementation. The act of effecting a plan. Activities include: teaching, monitoring, counseling, delegating, and coordinating.

Interdisciplinary. Reliant on the overlapping skills and knowledge of each team member and discipline, resulting in enhanced outcomes more comprehensive than the simple aggregation of the team members' individual efforts.

Intervention. A nursing activity that promotes health, assesses functional ability, helps clients to regain or improve coping abilities, implements planned strategies, and aims to prevent further disabilities.

ISONG. The International Society of Nurses in Genetics; the professional organization of and for nurses in genetics ranging from licensed graduate nurses credentialed in genetics to licensed nurses at all levels with an interest in genetics.

Multidisciplinary. Reliant on each team member or discipline contributing discipline-specific skills.

Outcome. An end result that is measurable, desirable, and observable, and translates into observable behaviors

Pedigree. A diagram of genetic relationships using standardized symbols and terminology, which typically spans a minimum of three generations; a comprehensive pedigree notes family members' medical history, noting individuals affected with, or at risk for, a genetic condition.

Pharmacogenomics. The study of genomic variations associated with drug response; often used interchangeably with **pharmacogenetics**, the study of allelic differences of single genes associated with individual variability in drug response.

Plan of care. Comprehensive outline of the steps that need to be completed to attain desired outcomes.

Predisposition. The presence of an allele, identified through molecular DNA analysis, that increases an individual's risk for developing a particular disorder or disease. The presence of the allele(s) does not assure that an individual will become affected, but places them at increased risk.

Presymptomatic. Not yet symptomatic, but carrying an allele, identified through molecular DNA analysis, that indicates that the person will eventually develop the associated disease or disorder.

Standard. An authoritative statement defined and promoted by the profession, by which the quality of practice, service, or education can be evaluated.

Transdisciplinary. Allowing team members to use skills learned from other disciplines, resulting in shared responsibility among team members for assessment, decision-making, and delivery of services.

APPENDIX A. STATEMENT ON THE SCOPE AND STANDARDS OF GENETICS CLINICAL NURSING PRACTICE (1998)

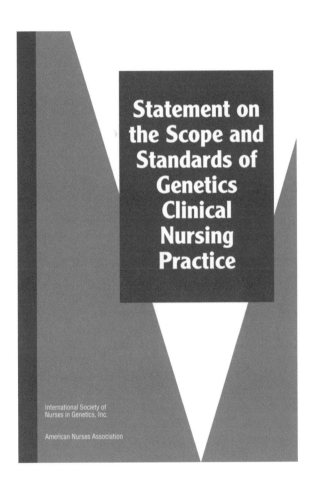

Statement on the Scope and Standards of Genetics Clinical Nursing Practice

International Society of Nurses in Genetics, Inc.

American Nurses Association

STATEMENT
on the
SCOPE and STANDARDS
of
Genetics Clinical
Nursing Practice

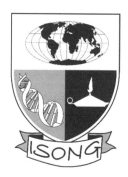

International Society of Nurses in Genetics, Inc.

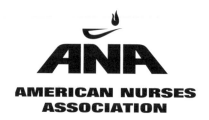

**AMERICAN NURSES
ASSOCIATION**

CONTENTS

INTRODUCTION

As the professional organization of nurses in genetics, the International Society of Nurses in Genetics, Inc., (ISONG) is responsible for defining and establishing the scope of professional nursing practice in genetics. In doing so, ISONG acknowledges the role of the American Nurses Association in defining the scope of practice for the nursing profession as a whole. ISONG supports the ANA *Nursing's Social Policy Statement* (ANA 1995), which charges specialty nursing organizations with defining their individual scope of practice and identifying the characteristics of their unique specialty area. In keeping with ISONG's responsibility, this document will begin with broad descriptions of genetics and nursing in genetics, followed by delineation of the scope of genetics clinical nursing practice.

Genetics

Basic and applied human genetics research defines, characterizes, and analyzes the hereditary basis for human variability, genetic conditions, their symptoms, population frequencies, and actual or potential therapies. Molecular and biochemical technology breakthroughs enhance clinical capabilities in diagnosing and treating genetic conditions. Likewise, advancements further the ability to predict susceptibility to and promote preventive therapies for genetically influenced chronic conditions such as cardiovascular and autoimmune diseases, cancer, and diabetes. The expanding human genetics field will continue to affect how genetics services are defined and delivered. These extend into an increasing variety of settings. Clinical genetics services include (1) ascertaining individuals, families, and populations needing genetics services; (2) providing and/or managing comprehensive care, which includes state-of-the-art genetics screening, diagnosis, counseling, and therapeutic modalities; (3) evaluating and improving genetics services; (4) educating individuals, families, and public and professional populations about genetics; and (5) assessing, deliberating, and developing recommendations for the ethical, legal, and social consequences of new and existing genetics services and technology.

Description of Genetics Nursing

All licensed registered nurses, regardless of their practice setting, have a role in the delivery of genetics services and the management of genetic information. Nurses require genetic knowledge to identify, refer, support, and care for persons affected by, or at risk for manifesting or transmitting, genetic conditions. As the public becomes more aware of the genetic contribution to health and disease, nurses in all areas of practice will be increasingly asked to address basic genetics-related questions, service needs, or both.

Genetics nursing is a separate clinical specialty that focuses on providing nursing care to clients who have known genetic conditions and/or birth defects, or who are at risk to develop them, or who have children with genetic conditions and/or birth defects. Genetic conditions are defined as variations, disorders, or diseases that are caused or influenced by genes and require nursing and/or medical intervention. For the purpose of this document, the term "genetic conditions" includes birth defects, which are abnormal conditions that range from minor to severe and result in debilitating disease, a physical or mental disability, or early death (March of Dimes 1994).

Genetics nursing practice may occur in any setting where clients affected by, or at risk for manifesting or transmitting, genetic conditions seek or are referred for genetic services. Genetics nursing involves an interpersonal relationship between the client and nurse. Clients are defined as (1) persons throughout the life span who have a genetic condition, (2) presymptomatic persons and families at risk for a genetic condition, (3) persons susceptible to diseases that have a genetic component, (4) couples at risk for having a child with a genetic condition, (5) persons or groups who need or request genetics information, and/or (6) groups, communities, or populations at risk for genetic conditions. Comprehensive genetics nursing practice is a dynamic process that involves interdisciplinary collegiality and collaboration or linkage with genetics professionals and other health care professionals to serve a shared mission of assisting clients in reaching their self-defined outcome. This outcome may be health education, improvement, maintenance, restoration, or a peaceful death.

Phenomena of Concern for Genetics Nursing Practice

The phenomena of concern to nurses are people's experiences with and responses to the health/illness continuum. The following is an illustrative, rather than comprehensive, list of client concerns or needs for which genetics nurses can develop methods of intervention and evaluation:

- Emotions related to discovery of and experiences with a genetic condition;
- Ethical, legal and social issues;
- Health education, improvement, maintenance, restoration, or a peaceful death;
- Incorporation of genetics knowledge into daily life;
- Informed decision making related to a genetic condition and the use of available genetics technology and services;
- Knowledge about risks for a genetic condition or chronic disease that has a genetic component and associated disability or morbidity;
- Participation in a complex health care system;
- Physiologic and pathophysiologic processes; and
- Self-image and self-esteem.

Theories Used in Genetics Nursing Practice

Genetics nurses use a number of theories for assessing, planning, implementing, and evaluating care that is responsive to nursing phenomena of concern. Such theories are derived from nursing, genetic, biologic, behavioral, and medical sciences, as well as other related fields. Theories provide a framework for understanding the phenomena of concern for nurses.

Genetics Nursing Practice Ethics

The *Code for Nurses with Interpretive Statements* (ANA 1985) is the foundation for ethical nursing practice and provides the basis for nursing practice in genetics. Sensitivity to cultural, lifestyle, racial, and ethnic diversity is integral in planning and providing services for clients with genetic conditions. The primary axiom of the profession is respect for individuals, and in this context the nurse supports the client's self-determination and autonomy.

Genetics Practice Settings for Nurses

Nurses may practice within health care settings that include, but are not limited to, hospitals and their affiliated clinics; regional genetics centers; community sites; state and federal agencies; private industry; and managed health care organizations. As genetics services continue to expand into a variety of settings, especially primary care settings, so too will genetics nursing practice.

Scope of Genetics Clinical Nursing Practice

Clinically applicable technology and information in the field of human genetics are rapidly expanding and affecting health care delivery. Nurses in all clinical settings will be increasingly relied upon to recognize and appropriately refer clients who can benefit from genetics services. To competently perform these functions, nurses should have a fundamental course in human genetics during their nursing preparation. In addition, didactic content and genetic experiences should be integrated into their clinical training. Practicing nurses who have not benefitted from such instruction should be encouraged to participate in continuing education programs that have genetic content, such as basic human genetics concepts, technological applications, and therapeutic modalities applicable to their specific clinical setting.

The scope of genetics nursing practice has two levels: basic and advanced. These levels of practice are distinguished by educational preparation, professional experience, practice focus, specific roles and functions, and certification. It is the responsibility of the nurse, professional nursing colleagues, and state boards of nursing to ensure that genetics nursing is practiced within the parameters of the individual's state nurse practice act and professional and ethical codes of nursing.

Basic Level

Although all nurses have occasion to care for clients who are affected with or at risk for conditions with a genetic component, basic level genetics nurses provide specific services on a routine basis to such clients and their families. Therefore, as a minimum, basic level genetics nurses must obtain didactic educational experience and ongoing continuing education as recommended for all nurses. In addition, basic level nurses require either formal genetics clinical experiences through their RN preparatory programs or on-the-job training in their specified role under the supervision of a professional trained in genetics. The nurse's knowledge and skill base is maintained through ongoing participation in genetics and nursing continuing education activities.

Genetics nursing practice at the basic level includes, but is not limited to, assessment, plan of care, intervention, and evaluation:

1. **Assessment.** Collecting and examining health data by participating in activities such as performing a physical examination; obtaining family, prenatal, and health histories; collecting appropriate laboratory data; inquiring into the client's desired health outcomes; and assessing the client's understanding of the genetic condition. This information is then used to develop nursing diagnoses and plan of care.

2. **Plan of Care.** Establishing an appropriate plan of nursing care designed for the client by collaborating with the client and coordinating that care with other health care professionals. Client-focused immediate and long-term health care goals are determined and used to develop a coordinated plan of action.

3. **Intervention.** Implementing interventions, which may include, but are not limited to, (1) heightening awareness about services and health behaviors that may reduce the risk or symptoms of a genetic condition; (2) facilitating successful adaptive responses to disease processes; (3) educating about, administering, and monitoring responses to therapies for a genetic condition; (4) advocating for and facilitating access to genetics resources and support groups; and (5) providing or reinforcing information about a genetic condition routinely cared for by the nurse.

4. **Evaluation.** Evaluating the plan of care, interventions, outcomes, and client's progress toward achieving mutually identified goals. When appropriate, the plan of care is adjusted on the basis of new data, resources, and the client's changing needs.

Advanced Level

Advanced nursing practice in genetics is administered by a licensed registered nurse who, at minimum, has (1) successfully completed an accredited graduate (master's or doctorate) program in nursing; (2) completed graduate-level genetics course work that includes human, molecular, biochemical, and population genetics content; technological applications; therapeutic modalities; and ethical, legal, and social implications of genetics information and technology; and (3) participated in genetics clinical training supervised by any combination of the following: (a) graduate nursing faculty, (b) genetics advanced practice nurse(s), and/or (c) board-certified geneticist(s). It is also expected that nurses at the advanced practice level possess current knowledge through participation in both advanced nursing and genetics continuing education activities. Documentation of these education and training activities will provide evidence of knowledge and expertise in genetics nursing. Genetics nursing certification, when it becomes available, will provide further evidence of the advanced practice nurse's expertise. Throughout this document, a nurse with a graduate degree in nursing who practices in genetics at the advanced practice level is referred to as a genetics advanced practice nurse (APN).

The critical elements that distinguish advanced from basic level genetics nursing practice are the complexity of decision making, leadership, the ability to negotiate complex organizations, and expanded practice skills and knowledge in nursing and genetics. Specialized knowledge about a wide variety of genetic conditions, technologies, and therapies enables the genetics APN to develop and/or provide innovative nursing care that is responsive to the client's diverse needs. Expanded skills may include, but are not limited to, pedigree construction; genetic physical assessment/dysmorphology examination; comprehensive, disease-specific health and family histories; interpretation of complex genetics laboratory data and test results; management of genetic therapeutic modalities; and genetic counseling. These skills augment the APN's ability to assess comprehensive health needs; develop diagnoses; plan, implement, and manage complex care; and evaluate outcomes of the care in collaboration with the client and a multidisciplinary team of health care professionals.

Beyond expansion of the basic level genetics nursing practice, the genetics APN provides consultation to nurses and other health care workers and seeks creative strategies to meet professional and public genetics education needs. Consultation services may include, but are not limited to, (1) participating in clinical evaluation of clients with genetic conditions, (2) guiding nurses and other health care professionals in the specialized care of clients with genetic conditions, (3) providing expert input into the development, management, and/or evaluation of nursing, medical, and interdisciplinary genetics clinical research projects, and (4) participating in assessment, deliberation, and development of recommendations for ethical, legal, and social consequences of existing and predicted genetics services and technologies. Educational interventions may include, but are not limited to, creating, producing, and evaluating educational materials and/or programs for professionals, clients, and the general population. A challenge for the genetics APN is to be active in the development of strategies for improving the basic genetics knowledge level of the more than 2 million practicing nurses in the United States, enabling them to participate in the identification, care, and referral of clients affected by, or at risk for manifesting or transmitting, genetic conditions. Furthermore, the genetics APN fosters growth and dissemination of genetics nursing knowledge by (1) participating in and/or conducting nursing research in genetics, (2) participating in multidisciplinary genetics research, and (3) presenting and publishing health care information related to genetics.

STANDARDS OF CARE

Introduction

Standards are authoritative statements in which the nursing profession describes the responsibilities for which nurses are accountable. The *Standards of Clinical Nursing Practice* (ANA 1991) was used as a foundation and framework for the genetics specialty standards in this booklet. The *Statement on the Scope and Standards of Genetics Clinical Nursing Practice* describes a competent level of professional nursing care and performance for nurses at both the basic and advanced levels of practice. With the exponential growth of knowledge and technological advances in genetics and the evolving role of nurses in this specialty area, these standards will need to be evaluated on an ongoing basis and revised as appropriate.

Standard I. Assessment

The client and the family affected by or at risk for a genetic condition are assessed by the genetics nurse to identify risk factors and intervention, information, service, and referral needs.

Measurement Criteria

1. Assessment begins with data collection through the use of interviews, observation, physical assessment, and formalized instruments.

2. Data collected may include, but are not limited to, the following:
   a. Biophysical status for which a dysmorphology examination and/or genetic laboratory testing may be used in addition to routine physical and laboratory testing;
   b. Client expectations;
   c. Coping and adaptation patterns;
   d. Cultural, community, and family support systems;
   e. Economic, environmental, and policy factors affecting the client's health;

f. Family history in pedigree format;
g. Family integrity, structure, and level of functioning;
h. Growth and development status;
i. Health beliefs and practices;
j. Medical histories;
k. Prenatal, perinatal, and neonatal histories;
l. Psychological status;
m. Spirituality; and
n. Values and beliefs.

3. Data collection identifies the following:
   a. Educational needs;
   b. Factors placing the client and/or family at increased risk for genetic conditions or birth defects;
   c. Short- and long-term goals, as well as follow-up needs;
   d. Individual and family strengths;
   e. The need for referral to other specialties, areas, or support groups;
   f. Nursing care needs;
   g. Risk factors associated with the genetic condition or birth defect; and
   h. Support systems.

4. Data are collected with consideration of client confidentiality from multiple sources, which may include, but are not limited to, the client, the family, other health care providers, past and current medical records, community sources, and social networks.

5. The assessment process and data analysis include discussion with the client and/or family about mutual health-related goals, roles, and responsibilities.

6. Ethical dimensions of practice such as confidentiality, informed consent, truth telling, disclosure, privacy, and nondiscrimination are integrated into the data collection and documentation process.

Standard II. Diagnosis

The genetics nurse analyzes the assessment data to determine diagnoses consistent with the nurse's education and state nurse practice act.

Measurement Criteria

1. Diagnoses and potential problem statements are derived from assessment data.

2. Diagnoses and risk factors are validated with the client, family, and other health professionals when appropriate and feasible.

3. Diagnoses identify actual or potential conditions or responses to genetic conditions or birth defects of clients pertaining to—
   a. Ethical, legal, and social implications;
   b. Health improvement, health maintenance, health restoration, or a peaceful death;
   c. Incorporation of genetics knowledge into routine daily life;
   d. Informed decision making related to a genetic condition, its management, and the use of available genetics technology and services;
   e. Knowledge and understanding about the risks for and associated with a genetic condition or chronic disease that has a genetic component;
   f. Participation in a complex health care system;
   g. Physiologic and pathophysiologic processes; and
   h. Psychosocial responses related to discovery of and experiences with a genetic condition.

4. Diagnoses and clinical impressions are documented in a manner that facilitates appropriate evaluations and the identification of client outcomes and their use in the plan of care and research.

Standard III. Outcome Identification

The genetics nurse identifies expected outcomes individualized to the client. Whenever possible, outcomes are identified in partnership with the client.

Measurement Criteria

1. Expected outcomes are derived from diagnoses.

2. Expected outcomes are documented as measurable goals.

3. Expected outcomes are formulated by the nurse and the client, significant others, and interdisciplinary team members, when feasible.

4. Expected outcomes are realistic in relation to the client's present and potential capabilities.

5. Expected outcomes are identified with consideration of the associated benefits and costs.

6. Expected outcomes estimate a time for attainment.

7. Expected outcomes provide direction for continuity of care.

8. Expected outcomes reflect current scientific knowledge in clinical application of human genetics.

9. Expected outcomes serve as a gauge for desired change in the client's health status.

10. Expected outcomes reflect awareness of and sensitivity to ethical, legal, and social issues.

Standard IV. Planning

The genetics nurse develops a plan of care that prescribes nursing interventions to attain expected outcomes. Whenever possible, the plan of care is developed in partnership with the client.

Measurement Criteria

1. The plan of care is individualized, tailored to the client's genetic condition or service needs, and it—
    a. Identifies appropriate interventions to achieve mutually identified, attainable goals;
    b. Specifies interventions that reflect current nursing practice, research, and genetics principles and counseling; and
    c. Provides mechanisms for consultation, referral, follow-up, and case management to ensure continuity of care.

2. The plan of care is developed in collaboration with the client, significant others, interdisciplinary team members, and community resources when appropriate and possible.

3. The plan of care is documented in a manner that allows accessibility by team members and modification of the plan as necessary.

4. The plan of care reflects awareness of and sensitivity to ethical, legal, and social issues.

Standard V. Implementation

The genetics nurse implements interventions identified in the plan of care.

Measurement Criteria

1. Interventions are based on the needs of the client and family and prudent nursing practice.

2. Interventions are consistent with the nurse's level of practice, education, certification, and state nurse practice act.

3. Interventions are consistent with the established plan of care.

4. Interventions are therapeutic and based on research.

5. Interventions are implemented in a safe, ethical, and appropriate manner and setting.

6. Interventions are validated with colleagues, the client, the family, and/or other support systems.

7. Interventions derived from the nursing plan of care are recorded in a systematic and standardized format.

8. Interventions adhere to principles of informed choice, truth telling, privacy, disclosure, confidentiality, and nondiscrimination.

Standard Va. Identification

The genetics nurse identifies individuals, families, groups, or communities with, or at risk for inheriting, manifesting, or transmitting, genetic conditions.

Measurement Criteria

1. Identification of an individual and/or family is based on assessment that may include genetic history, examination, and/or testing.

2. Identification of individuals, families, groups, and/or community is based on the ability to recognize genetic risk factors such as—
   a. Advanced reproductive age;
   b. Consanguinity;
   c. Family history of known or suspected genetic condition;
   d. High gene frequencies for specific groups and/or populations;
   e. Loss of attained developmental milestones;
   f. Mental retardation and/or birth defects of unknown etiology;
   g. Multiple miscarriages;
   h. Prenatal teratogens;
   i. Social, cultural, and ethnic health practices that may influence the manifestation of genetic conditions; and
   j. Stillbirth or neonatal death.

3. Identification is based on knowledge of human genetics principles.

4. Identification is based on knowledge of genetics services.

5. Identification is based on knowledge from current genetics and nursing research.

6. Identification is based on an awareness of, and sensitivity to, confidentiality, nondiscrimination, and the right not to know.

Standard Vb. Health Teaching

The genetics nurse promotes healthy patterns of living through health teaching.

Measurement Criteria

1. Health teaching is based on principles of learning.

2. Health teaching is provided on an individual, family, group, and/or community level.

3. Health teaching may focus on, but is not limited to, the following:
   a. Human/medical genetics principles;
   b. Complications related to genetic conditions, therapeutic modalities, and/or treatment effects;
   c. Health behaviors that may reduce either the risk for manifesting the genetic condition or the degree of morbidity and risk for premature death from an overt genetic condition;
   d. Resources for genetics information and services; and
   e. Up-to-date information related to genetic screening, testing, therapies, and research.

4. Health teaching methods are appropriate to the client's age, developmental level, education, gender, and ethnic–social background.

5. Health teaching includes constructive feedback and creative strategies to reinforce the client's learning.

6. Health teaching is evaluated and updated as needed, relative to current genetics and nursing information.

Standard Vc. Case Coordination

The genetics nurse coordinates or facilitates the coordination of health services to ensure continuity of care.

Measurement Criteria

1. Coordination of services is based on consideration of the client's physical, mental, emotional, and social health needs.

2. Coordination of services is provided with consideration of the client's right to privacy, confidentiality, and nondiscrimination.

3. Coordination of services is based on knowledge of the health care system and interdisciplinary communication principles and processes.

4. Coordination of services is provided in terms of the client's needs and accessibility, and the availability, quality, and cost-effectiveness of care.

5. Health-related services and more specialized care are obtained as needed from appropriate agencies and providers.

6. Genetic support groups or networking services are identified and offered.

7. The client's decisions related to the plan of care and treatment choices are respected and supported.

Standard Vd. Health Promotion and Health Maintenance

The genetics nurse implements strategies and interventions directed toward the promotion and maintenance of individual, family, group, and community health.

Measurement Criteria

1. Health promotion strategies are based on knowledge of—
   a. Epidemiological principles;
   b. Health beliefs, practices, and standards;
   c. Natural history of genetic conditions; and
   d. Social, cultural, and political issues that affect health.

2. Health promotion strategies are designed for clients identified as presymptomatic or at risk for inheriting, manifesting, or transmitting genetic conditions.

3. Community and genetics organizational resources are identified to assist consumers in using health promotion strategies.

Standard Ve. Psychosocial Counseling

The genetics nurse uses counseling interventions to assist clients in processing, adjusting to, and utilizing genetic information.

Measurement Criteria

1. Counseling is based on active listening and therapeutic communication skills.

2. Counseling is anticipatory, therapeutic, facilitative, supportive, and sensitive to client needs.

3. Counseling interventions (e.g., attachment or family integration promotion, coping enhancement, crisis intervention, decision-making support, and grief work facilitation) are documented.

4. The individual and/or family is referred to a mental health or social health care professional when counseling needs are determined to be beyond the skills of the genetics nurse.

Standard Vf. Genetic Therapeutics

The genetics nurse uses knowledge of genetic therapeutic interventions and applies clinical skills to restore the client's health and/or to prevent further disability.

1. Current knowledge of genetic therapeutic modalities (e.g., special diets, protein replacement therapy, transplantation, and somatic gene replacement therapy) are used to guide nursing actions.

2. The client's response to genetic therapeutic modalities is monitored, documented, and communicated to other health care professionals.

3. Nursing interventions are directed toward optimizing benefits and minimizing risks of side effects of genetic therapeutics, when possible.

4. Opportunities are provided for the client and/or family to question, discuss, and explore their feelings about past, current, and projected use of genetic therapeutic modalities.

Advanced Practice Interventions (Vg.–Vi.)

The following interventions (Standards Vg.–Vi.) may be performed only by the genetics advanced practice nurse.

Standard Vg. Genetic Counseling

The genetics advanced practice nurse uses counseling interventions to foster the client's and family's understanding about having or being at risk for inheriting, manifesting, or transmitting a genetic condition and promotes the client's and family's health adjustment to the information.

Measurement Criteria

1. Counseling is based on critical thinking, therapeutic principles, and advanced communication, interviewing, and crisis intervention techniques.

2. Counseling reinforces healthy physiologic and psychosocial behaviors and promotes a client-driven, informed decision-making process.

3. Counseling promotes client-driven, informed decision making by communicating information that may include, but is not limited to, the following:
   a. Clinical aspects of genetic conditions;
   b. Community and/or genetics organization resources and support services;
   c. Genetics concepts and principles;
   d. Potential complications of genetic conditions;
   e. Privacy, confidentiality, informed consent, truth telling,

disclosure, and nondiscrimination issues;

f. Risk assessment process and results;

g. Screening and diagnostic capabilities and results; and

h. Therapeutic and/or management options.

4. Counseling timing and follow-up needs are mutually determined with the client.

Standard Vh. Case Management

The genetics advanced practice nurse provides and/or facilitates case management for clients with, or at risk for manifesting, genetic conditions who have complex health care needs.

Measurement Criteria

1. Case management services are based on a comprehensive approach toward the client's physical, mental, emotional, and social health needs.

2. Case management services are based on the mutual rights, options, and responsibilities of the client and/or family.

3. Case management services are provided in terms of the client's needs and the accessibility, availability, quality, and cost-effectiveness of care.

4. Case management services are provided with respect for the client's rights to privacy, confidentiality, informed consent, truth telling, disclosure, and nondiscrimination.

5. Specialty and community health services are obtained as needed from the appropriate providers and agencies.

6. Continued relationships with agencies and providers are maintained throughout the client's use of the health care services to ensure continuity of care.

7. The client's decisions about the plan of care and treatment choices are respected.

Standard Vi. Consultation

The genetics advanced practice nurse provides consultation to the client and family, community, nurses, and/or other health care providers to enhance the plan of care and/or the abilities of others to provide appropriate care to individuals and families with genetic conditions.

Measurement Criteria

1. Consultation activities are based on knowledge of consultation models, communication and interviewing techniques, interdisciplinary team work, problem-solving skills, change and system theories, and other theories as indicated.

2. Consultation activities promote health and facilitate management for persons or groups with, or at risk for, a genetic condition.

3. A working alliance is established with the consultee on the basis of mutual respect and role responsibilities.

4. The decision to implement the plan of care or system change remains the responsibility of the consultee.

5. Consultation activities promote awareness and discussion of ethical dimensions such as privacy, confidentiality, informed consent, truth telling, disclosure, and nondiscrimination.

Standard VI. Evaluation

The genetics nurse evaluates the progress of the client and family toward attainment of outcomes.

Measurement Criteria

1. Evaluation is systematic and ongoing.

2. The client, family, and team members are involved in the evaluation process, as possible, to ascertain the client's level of satisfaction with and responses to care, and to evaluate the costs and benefits associated with the treatment process.

3. Evaluation reflects awareness of and sensitivity to ethical, legal, and social issues.

4. The client's condition and responses are recorded in a systematic and standardized format.

5. The effectiveness of interventions is evaluated relative to outcomes.

6. Ongoing assessment data are used to revise diagnoses, outcomes, and plan of care, as needed.

7. Revisions in diagnoses, outcomes, and plan of care are documented.

8. The revised plan provides for continuity of care and measurements for future evaluations.

STANDARDS OF PROFESSIONAL PERFORMANCE

Standard I. Quality of Care

The genetics nurse systematically evaluates the quality of care and the effectiveness of genetics nursing practice.

Measurement Criteria

The genetics nurse—

1. Participates in quality assessment and improvement activities as appropriate to position, education, and practice setting. These activities may include, but are not limited to, the following:
   a. Identifying areas of, and measurements for, improvement;
   b. Selecting effectiveness indicators for care delivery;
   c. Collecting and analyzing data; and
   d. Formulating recommendations to improve genetics nursing practice and client outcomes.

2. Seeks participation and input from the client in quality assessment and improvement activities.

3. Uses results from quality assessment and improvement activities to initiate changes in genetics nursing practice and genetic services, as appropriate.

4. Documents results of quality assessment and improvement activities.

Standard II. Performance Appraisal

The genetics nurse evaluates his or her own genetics nursing practice in relationship to professional practice standards and relevant statutes and regulations.

Measurement Criteria

The genetics nurse—

1. Performs appraisal of clinical practice and role performance to identify areas of competence and areas of developmental need.

2. Seeks and utilizes constructive input regarding clinical practice and role performance from peers, professional colleagues, clients, and others.

3. Develops plans to achieve goals identified through performance appraisal and review to enhance clinical practice and role performance.

4. Participates in peer review activities when possible.

Standard III. Education

The genetics nurse acquires and maintains current knowledge in his or her field of nursing practice and in clinically applicable genetics sciences.

Measurement Criteria

The genetics nurse—

1. Participates in educational activities to improve clinical and scientific knowledge in nursing and genetics and to increase knowledge of professional issues.

2. Seeks genetics nursing experiences and learning opportunities to maintain and enhance clinical and professional skills.

3. Participates in professional and interdisciplinary educational programs and activities.

4. Documents educational activities.

5. Seeks certification appropriate to genetics nursing role when available.

Standard IV. Collegiality

The genetics nurse contributes to the professional development of peers, colleagues, and others.

Measurement Criteria

The genetics nurse—

1. Uses practice opportunities to exchange knowledge, skills, and clinical observations with colleagues.

2. Provides mentoring as related to clinical practice, professional role responsibilities, and professional education and development.

3. Uses appropriate strategies to promote and maintain professional commitment toward self, clients, and other health care professionals.

4. Supports and facilitates clinical education of students in health professions.

5. Promotes mechanisms and opportunities for role-appropriate genetics education and certification.

6. Documents education activities.

Standard V. Ethics

The genetics nurse employs an ethical framework in professional decision making and in interactions with or on behalf of clients.

Measurement Criteria

The genetics nurse—

1. Is guided by the American Nurses Association *Code for Nurses with Interpretive Statements* (ANA 1985).

2. Provides care and services in a manner that preserves and protects client autonomy, dignity, and rights.

3. Adheres to the principles of informed choice, truth telling, disclosure, privacy, nondiscrimination, and confidentiality.

4. Functions as a client advocate.

5. Provides information, care, and services in an objective, nonjudgmental, and nondiscriminatory manner.

6. Identifies ethical dilemmas that occur within clinical practice and utilizes resources in formulating ethical responses.

7. Participates in formulating guidelines about the ethical considerations of new and existing genetic services and technology.

8. Reports unethical behavior, illegal acts, and abuse of client's rights to the appropriate institutional, licensing, and/or professional organization.

9. Is sensitive to and acts, when possible, to change institutional policies that foster moral distress in health care providers and clients.

10. Uses client's own language and level of communication to promote understanding of ethical issues.

11. Works with institutional and/or professional resources regarding ethical factors that may lead to internal and/or professional role conflict.

Standard VI. Collaboration

The genetics nurse collaborates with the client, significant others, and other health care providers in delivery of care and services.

Measurement Criteria

The genetics nurse—

1. Collaborates with clients, significant others, and health care providers in the formulation of goals, plans, and decisions related to care and provision of genetics services.

2. Consults with other health care providers to facilitate client care.

3. Makes referrals as needed while maintaining continuity of care.

Standard VII. Resource Utilization

The genetics nurse incorporates appropriate, efficient, and cost-effective resource utilization in planning and providing client care and services.

Measurement Criteria

The genetics nurse—

1. Discusses benefits, limitations, and cost-effectiveness of treatment options with the client, and when appropriate, the family.

2. Presents to the client and family factors related to safety, effectiveness, and cost when two or more clinical options would result in the same expected outcome.

3. Assists the client and family in identifying and securing available, appropriate services.

4. Participates in ongoing resource utilization review.

Standard VIII. Research

The genetics nurse contributes to the development and dissemination of genetics nursing knowledge through the use of research.

Measurement Criteria

The genetics nurse—

1. Uses interventions substantiated by research as appropriate to the nurse's position, education, and practice environment.

2. Conducts and/or participates in research as appropriate to the nurse's position, education, and practice environment. Such activities may include, but are not limited to, the following:
   a. Applying research findings to genetics nursing practice and assisting others in doing so;
   b. Consulting with research experts and colleagues as necessary;
   c. Critiquing research for application to genetics nursing practice;
   d. Developing, conducting, and/or evaluating genetics nursing research;
   e. Disseminating research results at professional meetings and through publication;
   f. Identifying clinical problems suitable for genetics nursing research;
   g. Participating in data collection;
   h. Participating in hospital, organization, or community-based research committees or programs;

     i.   Participating in multidisciplinary genetics research;

    j.   Sharing research activities with others; and

    k.   Using research findings in the development of policies, procedures, and guidelines for genetic client care.

3. Participates in human subject protection activities as appropriate and is particularly cognizant of the needs of the genetic client group served.

REFERENCES

American Nurses Association. 1995. *Nursing's Social Policy Statement*. Washington, DC: American Nurses Association.

American Nurses Association. 1991. *Standards of Clinical Nursing Practice*. Washington, DC: American Nurses Association.

American Nurses Association. 1985. *Code for Nurses with Interpretive Statements*. Washington, DC: American Nurses Association.

March of Dimes Birth Defects Foundation. 1994. *Birth Defects*. White Plains, NY: March of Dimes Birth Defects Foundation.

GLOSSARY

Assessment—The systematic process of collecting relevant client data for the purpose of determining actual or potential health problems and functional status. Methods used to obtain data include interviews, observations, physical examinations, review of records, collaboration with colleagues, and consideration of applicable literature and research.

Birth defect—Abnormal congenital condition ranging from minor to severe that may result in debilitating disease, a physical or mental disability, or early death. Birth defects may or may not have a genetic cause.

Case management—An intervention in which planned health care is integrated, coordinated, and advocated for individuals, families, and groups who require services. The purpose of case management is to decrease fragmentation and ensure access to appropriate, individualized, and cost-effective care. As a case manager, the nurse has the authority and accountability required to negotiate with multiple providers and to obtain diverse services for the benefit of persons with, or at risk for, genetic conditions.

Certification—The formal process by which clinical competence is validated in a specialty area of practice, typically involving examination of the applicant's knowledge.

Client—(1) A person who has or a couple with a child who has a genetic condition; (2) a presymptomatic person or family at risk for a genetic condition; (3) a person who is susceptible to a disease that has a genetic component; (4) a person or couple who is at risk for having a child with a genetic condition; (5) a person or group who needs or requests genetic information; or (6) a group, community, or population that has or is at risk for genetic conditions.

Comprehensive genetics nursing practice—A dynamic process that involves interdisciplinary collegiality and collaboration or linkage with other genetic and health care professionals to serve a shared mission of assisting clients in reaching their self-defined outcome. This outcome may be health education, improvement, maintenance, or restoration, or a peaceful death.

Congenital—Present at birth. Congenital anomalies may or may not be genetic.

Consanguinity—Relationship by descent from a common ancestor. A union between two persons who are first-, second-, or third-degree relatives is at a significantly increased risk for having offspring with a recessive genetic condition than an unrelated couple.

Crisis intervention—A short-term therapeutic process that focuses on the rapid resolution of an immediate need or emergency using available personal, family, and/or environmental resources.

Dysmorphology—The study of abnormal physical development (e.g., as might be found in a syndrome).

Evaluation—The process of determining both the client's progress toward attainment of expected outcomes and the effectiveness of nursing care.

Gene frequency—The number of individuals with a particular allele (form of a gene) in a specified population divided by the total specified population.

Gene replacement therapy—Replacement of an abnormally functioning gene with a normally functioning gene for the purpose of correcting or preventing a genetic disease.

Genetic condition—Variations, disorders, birth defects, or diseases that are caused or influenced by genes and may or may not be transmitted from parent to offspring.

Genetic counseling—A process of information exchange between genetics health care professionals and individuals or families. The genetics health care professional seeks to impartially provide comprehensive information regarding the medical facts of and expectations for the course of the disorder, mode of inheritance, recurrence risks, and diagnostic and treatment options, and to promote adjustment and provide support for the client's chosen course of action.

Genetic diagnosis—Cytogenetic, biochemical, or molecular studies, and/or identification of a clinical phenotype that identifies the individual as having a genetic condition.

Genetic screening—Testing that refines the calculation of an individual's risk of manifesting or transmitting a genetic condition or having offspring with a birth defect. Types of genetic screening include neonatal screening, prenatal screening, and population screening. Effective screening programs meet specific criteria: (1) the genetic condition is relatively frequent in a population; (2) the test is highly sensitive, specific, and relatively inexpensive; (3) the benefits of the program outweigh its psychological, social, ethical, or economic costs; (4) the screening test results can be confirmed by diagnostic tests in a timely manner; (5) treatment and/or reproductive options are available for individuals testing positive; and (6) appropriate counseling and support services are available for person(s) identified as being at risk for manifesting or transmitting genetic conditions or having offspring with a birth defect.

Genetic therapeutic modalities—Treatment for a genetic disorder. These approaches include, but are not limited to, (1) dietary modification (e.g., for phenylketonuria and familial hypercholesterolemia); (2) replacement of defective gene (gene therapy) (e.g., for inherited immune deficiencies); (3) replacement of deficient enzyme (e.g., for Gaucher's disease); (4) other gene product replacement [e.g., as in hemophilias (factor VIII, IX)]; (5) other medical therapies (e.g., penicillamine for Wilson's disease or allopurinol for hyperuricemias); and (6) surgical approaches (e.g., renal transplantation for polycystic kidney disease).

Genetics advanced practice nurse (APN)—A nurse with a master's or higher degree in nursing with additional education and training in genetics who practices at the advanced practice level. Beyond expansion of the basic level genetics nursing practice, the genetics APN uses specialized knowledge to provide consultation to nurses and other health care workers and seeks creative strategies to meet professional and public genetics education needs. Furthermore, the genetics APN fosters growth and dissemination of genetics nursing knowledge through research, presenting, and publishing activities.

Genetics nursing—A separate clinical specialty that focuses on providing nursing care to clients who have or are at risk for developing genetic conditions and/or birth defects, or who have children with genetic conditions and/or birth defects.

Implementation—The act of effecting a plan that may include any or all of these activities: teaching, intervening, delegating, and coordinating. The client, significant others, or health care providers may be designated to implement interventions within the plan of care.

Interventions—Nursing activities that promote and foster health, assess functional ability, help clients to regain or improve their coping abilities, implement planned strategies, and aim to prevent further disabilities.

ISONG—The International Society of Nurses in Genetics, Inc., the professional organization of and for nurses in genetics ranging from licensed graduate nurses credentialed in genetics to licensed nurses at all levels with an interest in genetics.

Outcome—A planned result of interventions, which includes the degree of wellness and the continued need for care, medication, support, counseling, and education.

Pedigree—In medical genetics, a diagrammatic representation of a comprehensive family history, noting individuals affected with or at risk for a genetic condition and their relationship to the client.

Plan of care—Comprehensive outline of care to be delivered to attain desired outcomes.

Presymptomatic—Inherited gene alteration known to cause a condition that is genetically identified before the appearance of symptoms. For example, the altered gene for Huntington's disease can be detected through molecular testing before symptoms appear.

Registered nurse (RN)—An individual educationally prepared in nursing and licensed by the state board of nursing to practice nursing in that state. Registered nurses may qualify for specialty practice at two levels: basic and advanced. These levels are differentiated by educational preparation, professional experience, type of practice, and certification.

Scope of practice—A range of nursing functions and abilities that are differentiated according to level of practice, role of the nurse, and work setting. The parameters are determined by each state's nursing practice act, professional code of ethics, and nursing practice standards, as well as by each individual's personal competency to perform particular activities or functions.

Standard—Authoritative statement enunciated and promulgated by the profession to establish an expected quality of practice, service, or education.

Susceptible—The presence of an altered gene or genes identified through molecular DNA techniques that increase an individual's risk for developing a particular disorder or disease. The presence of the altered gene or genes does not ensure that an individual will become affected, but it places him or her at increased risk. Examples are some common multifactorial conditions, such as diabetes mellitus and some cancers.

Teratogen—A physical or chemical agent that is associated with an increased risk of birth defects.

INDEX

Pages in the 1998 *Statement on the Scope and Standards of Genetics Clinical Nursing Practice* are enclosed in brackets [ ].

Assessment (*continued*)
  evaluation and, [1998] 82
  identification and, [1998] 74
  planning and, 26
  standard of practice, 22
    [1998] 69–70
Association of Genetic Nurses and
    Counselors (AGNC), 8
Australia, 8

B
Basic genetics/genomics nursing
    practice, 12, 13
  [1998] 66–67
  assessment, 22
    [1998] 69–70
  case coordination, [1998] 76–77
  collaboration, 40
    [1998] 87
  collegiality, 39
    [1998] 85
  consultation, 31
  coordination of care, 28
  counseling, 33
  diagnosis, 23
    [1998] 71
  education, 37
    [1998] 84–85
  ethics, 41
    [1998] 85–86
  evaluation, 34
  genetic therapeutics, [1998] 78–79
  health promotion and health
    maintenance, [1998] 77
  health teaching, [1998] 75–76
  health teaching and health promotion,
    29
  identification, [1998] 74–75
  implementation, 27
    [1998] 73–74
  leadership, 47–48
  outcomes identification, 24
    [1998] 72
  performance appraisal, [1998] 83–84
  planning, 25
    [1998] 73
  prescriptive authority and treatment, 32

professional practice evaluation, 38
psychosocial counseling, [1998] 78
quality of care, [1998] 83
quality of practice, 35–36
research, 43
  [1998] 88–89
resource utilization, 45
  [1998] 87–88
Belgium, 8
Birth defect (defined), [1998] 91
Body of knowledge, 10
  [1998] 63, 64, 65, 67, 69
  education and, 37
    [1998] 84
  genetic counseling and, [1998] 79
  genetic therapeutics and, [1998] 78
  identification and, [1998] 75
  implementation and, 27
  outcomes identification and, 24
    [1998] 72
  quality of practice and, 35
  research and, 44
    [1998] 88
  See also Education of genetics/
    genomics nurses; Research

C
Canada, 5–6, 8
Canadian Association of Genetic
    Counsellors (CAGC), 5, 6
Canadian College of Medical Genetics,
    5
Canadian Nurses Association, 6
Care recipient. *See* Client
Care standards. *See* Standards of practice
Caregiver (defined), 53
Case coordination
  standard of practice, [1998] 76–77
  See also Case management;
    Coordination of care
Case management, [1998] 68
  defined, [1998] 91
  diagnosis and, [1998] 71
  planning and, [1998] 73
  standard of practice, [1998] 80–81
  See also Case coordination;
    Coordination of care

Case study in genetics/genomics nursing practice, 15–16
Certification and credentialing, 4, 5, 6, 8
  [1998] 65, 67
  advanced practice, 14
  basic practice, 13
  collegiality and, [1998] 85
  defined, 54
    [1998] 91
  education and, [1998] 85
  ethics and, [1998] 86
  genetics specialization, 16–17
  implementation and, [1998] 74
  leadership and, 47
  quality of practice and, 36
Certified Registered Nurse Anesthetist (CRNA), 14
Client
  [1998] 66, 67, 68
  assessment and, 22
    [1998] 69, 70
  case coordination and, [1998] 76, 77
  case management and, [1998] 80, 81
  collaboration and, 40
    [1998] 87
  collegiality and, 39
    [1998] 85
  consultation and, 31
    [1998] 81
  counseling and, 33
  defined, 9, 21, 53–54
    [1998] 63, 91
  diagnosis and, 23
    [1998] 71
  ethics and, 41
    [1998] 86
  evaluation and, 34
    [1998] 82
  genetic counseling and, [1998] 79, 80
  genetic therapeutics and, [1998] 79
  health promotion and health maintenance, [1998] 77
  health teaching and, [1998] 76
  identification and, [1998] 74
  implementation and, [1998] 74
  outcomes identification and, 24
    [1998] 72

  planning and, 25
    [1998] 73
  prescriptive authority and treatment, 32
  performance appraisal and, [1998] 84
  professional practice evaluation and, 38
  psychosocial counseling and, [1998] 78
  quality of care and, [1998] 83
  relationship with nurse, 9, 10, 41
  resource utilization and, 45
    [1998] 87, 88
  See also Education of clients and families; Family
Clinical Nurse Midwife (CNM), 14
Clinical Nurse Specialist (CNS), 14
Clinical settings. See Practice settings
Code of ethics (defined), 54
Code of Ethics for Nurses, 10, 41
Code of Ethics for Nurses with Interpretive Statements, 10, 41
    [1998] 64
  See also Ethics
Collaboration, 9
  [1998] 63, 66, 68
  implementation and, 27
  planning and, [1998] 73
  standard of professional performance, 40
    [1998] 87
  See aso Healthcare providers; Inter- disciplinary health care; Referrals
Collegiality, 9, 13
  [1998] 63, 65
  consultation and, 31
  diagnosis and, 23
  education and, 37
  implementation and, 27
    [1998] 74
  leadership and, 47
  performance appraisal and, [1998] 84
  professional practice evaluation and, 38
  research and, 43
    [1998] 88
  standard of professional performance, 39
    [1998] 85

Decision-making (*continued*)
diagnosis and, [1998] 71
ethics and, [1998] 85
genetic counseling and, [1998] 79
implementation and, [1998] 74
leadership and, 47, 48
research and, 43
Diagnosis, 2, 10, 11, 15, 16, 19
[1998] 66, 68
assessment and, 22
defined, 54
evaluation and, 34
[1998] 82
genetic counseling and, [1998] 80
outcomes identification and, [1998]
72
planning and, 25, 26
prescriptive authority and treatment,
32
standard of practice, 23
[1998] 71
Documentation
assessment and, 22
[1998] 70
collaboration and, 40
collegiality and, [1998] 85
coordination of care and, 28
counseling and, 33
diagnosis and, 23
[1998] 71
education and, 37
[1998] 85
evaluation and, 34
[1998] 82
genetic therapeutics and, [1998] 78
implementation and, 27
[1998] 74
outcomes identification and, 24
[1998] 72
planning and, 25
[1998] 73
psychosocial counseling and, [1998]
78
quality of practice and, 35, 36
[1998] 83
Dysmorphology (defined), 54
[1998] 92

Dysmorphology assessment (defined),
55

E
Economic issues. *See* Cost control
Education of genetics/genomics nurses,
4, 8, 10, 18
[1998] 65, 66, 67
advanced practice, 14, 15
basic practice, 13
collaboration and, 40
collegiality and, 39
[1998] 85
coordination of care and, 28
diagnosis and, [1998] 71
implementation and, [1998] 74
international, 5, 6, 7, 8
quality of care and, [1998] 83
research and, 43
[1998] 88
standard of professional performance,
37
[1998] 84–85
See also Mentoring; Professional
development
Education of clients and families, 2
[1998] 63, 64, 66, 68
assessment and, [1998] 70
counseling and, 33
resource utilization and, 45
See also Family; Health promotion
and health maintenance; Health
promotion; Health teaching and
health promotion
Environmental interactions, 1, 3, 9, 12, 19
assessment and, 22
coordination of care and, 28
Ethics, 2, 10, 14
[1998] 64, 67, 68
assessment and, [1998] 70
consultation and, 31
[1998] 81
diagnosis and, [1998] 71
evaluation and, 34
[1998] 82
implementation and, [1998] 74
outcomes identification and, [1998] 72

planning and, [1998] 73
quality of practice and, 35
research and, 43
  [1998] 89
standard of professional performance,
  41–42
  [1998] 85–86
See also Code of Ethics for Nurses
  with Interpretive Statements;
  Laws, statutes, and regulations
Evaluation, 10, 11, 12, 13
  [1998] 66, 67, 68
defined, 55
  [1998] 92
diagnosis and, [1998] 71
health teaching and health promotion,
  29
  [1998] 76
resource utilization and, 45, 46
standard of practice, 34
  [1998] 82
Evidence-based practice, 9, 12
assessment and, 22
consultation and, 31
counseling and, 33
defined, 55
education and, 37
health teaching and health promotion,
  29
implementation and, 27
leadership and, 48
outcomes identification and, 24
planning and, 25
prescriptive authority and treatment,
  32
quality of practice and, 36
See also Research
Expected outcomes (defined), 55

F

Family, 2, 13, 15, 19
assessment and, 22
  [1998] 69, 70
case management and, [1998] 80
collaboration and, 40
  [1998] 87
consultation and, [1998] 81

defined, 55
diagnosis and, 23
  [1998] 71
evaluation and, 34
  [1998] 82
genetic counseling and, [1998] 79
genetic therapeutics and, [1998] 79
health promotion and health
  maintenance, [1998] 77
health teaching and, [1998] 76
identification and, [1998] 74
implementation and, [1998] 74
outcomes identification and, 24
  [1998] 72
planning and, 25
  [1998] 73
prescriptive authority and treatment,
  32
psychosocial counseling and, [1998] 78
resource utilization and, 45
  [1998] 87, 88
See also Client; Education of clients
  and families
Family history, 12, 15, 18
  [1998] 66, 67
assessment and, [1998] 70
See also Data collection; Pedigree
Financial issues. *See* Cost control

G

Gene (defined), 55
Gene frequency (defined), [1998] 92
Gene replacement therapy (defined),
  [1998] 92
Genetic condition, 9, 15, 19
  [1998] 64
defined, 55
  [1998] 63, 92
See also Single-gene disorders
Genetic diagnosis (defined), [1998] 93
Genetic Diseases Act (1976), 3
Genetic Nurses Network, 4
Genetic Nursing Committee of Japan,
  6–7
Genetic Nursing Credentialing
  Commission (GNCC), 5, 6, 16–17
See also Certification and credentialing

Genetic predisposition (defined), 55
Genetic screening (defined), [1998] 93
Genetic testing, 11, 12
  assessment and, 22
    [1998] 69
  counseling and, 33
  defined, 55
  ethics and, 42
  health teaching and, [1998] 76
  identification and, [1998] 74
  prescriptive authority and treatment,
    32
Genetic therapeutics
  defined, [1998] 93
  standard of practice, [1998] 78–79
Genetics, 1–2
  [1998] 62
  defined, 1, 55
  See also Genomics
Genetics centers, 5, 11
Genetics Clinical Nurse (GCN), 17
  defined, 56
Genetics counseling, 4, 5, 6, 11, 12
  [1998] 68
  defined, 56
    [1998] 92–93
  standard of practice, [1998] 79–80
Genetics nurse in advanced practice
    (defined), 13, 15
  [1998] 67, 93–94
  See also Advanced genetics/genomics
    nursing practice
Genetics nursing practice (defined), 56
  [1998] 63, 94
Genetics services, 2, 4
  [1998] 62, 65
Genetics/genomics nursing
  advanced practice, 11–12, 13–15, 16
    [1998] 67–68
  Australia, 8
  basic practice, 12, 13
    [1998] 66–67
  Belgium, 8
  body of knowledge, 10, 24, 27, 35, 37,
    44
    [1998] 63, 64, 65, 67, 69, 72, 75, 78, 79,
    84, 88

Canada, 5–6, 8
case study, 15–16
certification, 4, 5, 6, 8
characteristics, 2–3, 8–11
  [1998] 63–65
defined, 2–3, 56
education, 4, 5, 6, 7, 8, 10, 13, 14, 15,
  18, 28, 37, 39, 40, 43
  [1998] 65, 66, 67, 71, 74, 83, 84–85, 88
essential attributes, 10–11
history, 1–2, 3–8
Japan, 6–7
Netherlands, 8
New Zealand, 8
relationship with client, 9, 10, 41
roles, 2, 8–9, 12–15
scope of practice, 1–19
  [1998] 62–68
standards of practice, 22–34
  [1998] 69–82
standards of professional performance,
  35–48
  [1998] 83–89
trends, 17–19
United Kingdom, 7–8, 18
United States, 3–5, 6, 8, 14, 16, 17, 18
Genomics, 1–2, 19
  defined, 1, 56
  See also Genetics
Genomics Policy Unit, 18
Guidelines
  assessment and, 22
  ethics and, 41
    [1998] 86
  leadership and, 48
  research and, 43
    [1998] 89
  See also Standards of practice;
    Standards of professional
    performance

H
Health (defined), 56
Health promotion and health
    maintenance
  consultation and, [1998] 81
  diagnosis and, [1998] 71

Interventions (*continued*)
evaluation and, 34
[1998] 82
genetic counseling and, [1998] 79
genetic therapeutics and, [1998] 79
health promotion and health
maintenance, [1998] 77
implementation and, [1998] 73, 74
planning and, 26
[1998] 73
psychosocial counseling and, [1998] 78
research and, [1998] 88

J
Japan, 6–7
Japan Academy of Nursing, 7
Japan Nurses Association, 7

K
Knowledge base. *See* Body of knowledge

L
Laws, statutes, and regulations, 2, 8, 10,
13, 14
[1998] 64, 67, 68
diagnosis and, [1998] 71
evaluation and, 34
[1998] 82
implementation and, [1998] 74
outcomes identification and, [1998]
72
planning and, 25
[1998] 73
prescriptive authority and treatment,
32
performance appraisal and, [1998] 83
professional practice evaluation and,
38
See also Ethics
Leadership, 13
[1998] 67
collaboration and, 40
coordination of care and, 28
standard of professional
performance,
Levels of genetics/genomics nursing
practice, 12–15

[1998] 65–68
See also Advanced genetics nursing
practice; Basic genetics nursing
practice
Licensing. *See* Certification and
credentialing

M
Measurement criteria. *See* Criteria
Mentoring, 45
collegiality and, 39
[1998] 85
leadership and, 47
Multidisciplinary healthcare (defined), 57
See also Interdisciplinary health care

N
National Coalition for Health
Professional Education in Genetics
(NCHPEG), 18
National Health Service, 7
Netherlands, 8
New Zealand, 8
Nurse practitioner (NP), 14
Nursing care standards. *See* Standards
of care
Nursing standards. *See* Standards of
practice; Standards of professional
performance

O
Outcomes, 13
[1998] 66, 67, 68
collaboration and, 40
defined, 57
[1998] 94
diagnosis and, 23
[1998] 71
ethics and, 41, 42
evaluation and, 34
[1998] 82
planning and, 25
[1998] 73
quality of practice and, 35
resource utilization and, 45
[1998] 87
See also Outcomes identification